KUNG FU is the fascinating Chinese style of karate which can be practiced alone or with a partner. It is one of the earliest stylized forms of the ancient exotic Oriental fighting arts.

TAI CHI is the classical system of Chinese exercise. Still practiced in China today, tai chi is a wonderful solo exercise to maintain body flexibility, develop body consciousness and promote good body movement through body awareness.

BRUCE TEGNER explains and teaches kung fu and tai chi in clear and intelligent terms which the Western reader can easily understand and follow. Every routine is illustrated with distinct photos and precise text.

"... Mr. Tegner offers his customary informed commentary ... without oversimplifying or misrepresenting either art. The book is recommended for physical fitness collections."

LIBRARY JOURNAL

BRUCE TEGNER is an authority in the field of weaponless fighting and related skills for sport, recreation, physical fitness and self-defense. He is regarded as this country's outstanding teacher, writer and innovator in the subject field.

In this field, in which most individuals study only one narrow specialty, Mr. Tegner's background is unusual and covers a wide range of the arts. Both his parents were professional teachers of judo and jiu jitsu and they began his training when he was only two years old! His mother and father taught him the fundamentals; Oriental and European experts instructed him from the age of eight. His education covered many aspects of weaponless, sword and stick fighting techniques. At the age of 20 he was the California state judo champion. He holds black belts in karate and judo.

Although Bruce Tegner was trained in the traditional manner, he originated a new style and method when he began to teach. He separated and distinguished between sport and self-defense forms of weaponless fighting. He introduced new concepts for modern applications of the ancient skills.

In the U.S. armed forces, Mr. Tegner trained instructors to teach weaponless combat, he taught military police tactics and he coached sport judo teams. He has trained actors and devised fight scenes for films and TV. From 1952 to 1967 he operated his own school in Hollywood where he taught men, women and children, exceptionally gifted students and blind and disabled persons.

He has developed a special course of weaponless defense and control for law enforcement, which he teaches in the Police Science Department of Moorpark College in California. With Alice McGrath, he has developed special, original courses of self-defense suitable for inclusion in physical education classes at secondary school level; the texts for these courses have been widely adopted. Together, Mr. Tegner and Miss McGrath are engaged in a teacher-training program, through California Lutheran College, which prepares physical education teachers to teach basic self-defense to boys and men and girls and women.

Bruce Tegner has twenty-five books in print with additional titles in preparation.

BOOKS BY BRUCE TEGNER

* COMPLETE BOOK OF KARATE

* COMPLETE BOOK OF JUDO

COMPLETE BOOK OF JUKADO: JIU JITSU

COMPLETE BOOK OF AIKIDO and HOLDS & LOCKS

* SELF-DEFENSE FOR BOYS & MEN (A Physical Education Course)

SELF-DEFENSE FOR GIRLS & WOMEN [with Alice McGrath] (A Physical Education Course)

SELF-DEFENSE FOR WOMEN [with Alice McGrath] A Simple Method for Home Study

SELF-DEFENSE YOU CAN TEACH YOUR BOY: A Confidence-Building Course (elementary school age)

KARATE: The Open Hand and Foot Fighting

KARATE: Volume Two, Traditional Sport Forms

SAVATE: French Foot and Fist Fighting

BRUCE TEGNER METHOD OF SELF-DEFENSE

JUDO FOR FUN: Sport Techniques

AIKIDO and Jiu Jitsu Holds & Locks

JUDO & KARATE BELT DEGREES: Requirements, Rules

KARATE & JUDO EXERCISES

BLACK BELT JUDO, KARATE, JUKADO

* KUNG FU & TAI CHI: Chinese Karate & Classical Exercise

SELF-DEFENSE NERVE CENTERS & PRESSURE POINTS

DEFENSE TACTICS FOR LAW ENFORCMENT: Volume One, Weaponless Defense & Control

STICK FIGHTING: SELF-DEFENSE

Additional titles in preparation

* **Published by Bantam Books**

KUNG FU
& TAI CHI

CHINESE KARATE AND
CLASSICAL EXERCISES

by

BRUCE TEGNER

BANTAM BOOKS

TORONTO · NEW YORK · LONDON

KUNG FU & TAI CHI:
Chinese Karate & Classical Exercises
by BRUCE TEGNER

A Bantam Book/Published by arrangement with
Thor Publishing Company

Thor edition published February 1968
2nd printing September 1969
3rd printing April 1972
4th printing January 1973

Bantam edition published June 1973
2nd printing
3rd printing

Manuscript prepared under the supervision of
ALICE McGRATH

Published simultaneously in the United States and Canada

Bantam Books are published by Bantam Books, Inc., a National General company. Its trade-mark, consisting of the words "Bantam Books" and the portrayal of a bantam, is registered in the United States Patent Office and in other countries. Marca Registrada. Bantam Books, Inc., 666 Fifth Avenue, New York, N.Y. 10019.

PRINTED IN THE UNITED STATES OF AMERICA

APPRECIATION:

To V. E. CHRISTENSEN, M.D., the author wishes
to extend grateful thanks. Dr. Christensen generously
devoted time and effort in research for this book
and he demonstrates the techniques in the
photos. He is assisted in the two-man forms by
Herk Rossilli, whose cooperation is appreciated.
Helen and Don Phillips were helpful in many ways.

The teachings of YANG CHU (fl. 4th century B.C.)

In the fourth century B.C., the Chinese
philosopher Yang Chu presented a new
philosophical concept—the concept of
naturalism as a way of fulfillment of
human life. Observing that man lacks sharp
teeth and claws, thick fur and feathers,
he concluded that man must develop his
own strengths, rather than imitate those of
the beasts. Man's intelligence, said Yang Chu,
distinguishes man from beast. Prowess, which
is natural in beasts, is despicable in man.
Man must find the way which is natural for him.
Yang Chu taught that the man who tries to find
his nature in the nature of beasts, loses his
nature as a man. The naturalism which Yang Chu
proposed was not the naturalism of animals, but
the naturalism of human creatures.

CONTENTS

FOREWORD

BRUCE TEGNER occupies a position unique in the field of Oriental fighting skills; he is both advocate and adversary; he is both innovator and preserver of the ancient arts. It is symbolic of his special position as a teacher of karate, judo, jiu jitsu and related skills, that he is regarded as an eminent authority in this field by such diverse journals as the JAPAN TIMES and SCHOLASTIC COACH.

Modern physical educators have had, until very recently, a resistance to incorporating the Oriental fighting skills into programs for health, exercise and recreation. Traditionalists in the field of Oriental fighting skills have had a resistance to any change in their specialties which would bring these activities more into line with modern concepts of health and physical education. Bruce Tegner's efforts to bring the two opposites into some understanding of the virtues and values of each, have been remarkably successful.

The fundamental proposition which Bruce Tegner puts forward is this: that the physical activity of kung fu, judo, aikido, etc, is not bound to the superstitions and archaic social attitudes which surround them. It is these superstitions and anti-social concepts which have been a barrier to evaluating the basic physical activity camouflaged by the mysticism. A teacher of physical education feels repugnance, and rightfully so, when he is told that kung fu training prepares one to kill his adversary with a mere poke of the finger at the right time of day. His objections are social, moral and anatomical.

Even if it were possible to learn the "deadly" art of
finger-poking, physical education teachers and
recreation directors would hardly be expected to
approve of it, any more than they would be expected
to approve of fencing practice in which the blades
were sharpened and the opponents made "points"
by inflicting injury.

A comparison of judo and kung fu is useful here.
Though judo is a relatively modern game (it was
invented at the end of the last century in Japan, just
about the time volleyball was invented in the United
States) it did not, until very recent years shake off
the covering of mysticism and ceremony which
obscured the excellent physical activity. Though judo
was practiced as a sport, it was talked about as though
it were a religion. Though judo was intended for
physical development, it was overwhelmed with
ceremonial practices and ancient Japanese cultural
appendages. The Japanese player of judo was expected to observe Japanese cultural and social customs
in his practice of judo, not because it was inherent
in the game, but because it was inherent in his
society. There never was any reason why the non-
Japanese person practicing judo should be required
to bow to the Shinto shrine before beginning his play!
The social customs were exported with the physical
activity and the two were mingled to the delight of
the cultists and the dismay of physical educators.

The fad for judo as a "way of life", the fad for judo
as a facet of purely Japanese culture, the fad for
judo as self-defense, all these fads have passed,
pretty much, and we are left with the physical activity of judo, which, it turns out is a marvelous sport
and perfectly suitable for recreation, physical fit-

ness, and pastime activity. For the highly serious sports player, it can be followed all the way up to Olympic competition.

This is not to suggest that kung fu is on its way to becoming an Olympic sport, but it is a reminder that separation from old cultural connections does not diminish a physical activity; it can, on the contrary, give it new life.

In this presentation of kung fu and tai chi, Bruce Tegner shows all the ancient movements which can be practiced for health and pleasure, without suggesting that we need to relinquish a rational view of the world or ourselves. He does not ask us to accept kung fu as modern, practical self-defense, but as an interesting and satisfying body exercise. He does not make the claim that tai chi is superior to all other forms of exercise; he suggests that it is a marvelous and beautiful form of exercise for which no exaggerated claims need be made.

Just as archery, fencing, kayaking and riding are practiced for physical fitness and recreation, without having to justify them in terms of combat or transportation, so kung fu and tai chi may be separated from their archaic origins and practiced with delight, says Bruce Tegner, and many individuals, particularly physical educators, will find themselves in enthusiastic agreement.

A LETTER TO MY READER-STUDENTS

This letter is directed to those of you who have no source of information or instruction except that which you find in books. Indeed, this book was written in direct response to requests made for it by reader-students.

I would like to express my appreciation to the many people who have accepted my books so warmly. I greatly appreciate the letters you send and you may be assured that I read them all carefully. Because I cannot make separate replies to so many letters and inquiries, I am taking this opportunity to answer the most-frequently asked questions, instead of writing the usual introduction. Following are the questions which are asked most often:

HOW IS KUNG FU (OR GUNG FU) DIFFERENT?

Kung fu, also known as gung fu, is the older, Chinese style of karate, probably derived from an even older style of hand and foot fighting which originated in India. The hand and foot blows of *all* styles of karate are similar. If you look at photos of any style of karate you will see the same types of hand blows and the same types of kicking blows. The principal differences between kung fu and other styles of karate are: a preference for clawing, stabbing hand blows and a different, stylistic manner of practicing the routines (or forms).

However, it is not correct to speak of kung fu as though it were one, well-defined style of karate, for within kung fu there are two main divisions and a number of subdivisions with respect to types of blows preferred, style of practice and general attitude toward the material. The hard-style kung fu systems show a clear preference for strength and power techniques, an inclination toward use of the kicks and an emphasis on hand conditioning.

Soft-style kung fu emphasizes speed, rather than power, emphasizes hand blows in preference to foot blows, and prefers to hit at vulnerable body targets.

WHAT IS THE IRON HAND?

The iron hand is a very heavily conditioned hand, favored in hard-style kung fu and also used in other hard-style karate systems, including the Hawaiian, some Japanese and some Korean systems.

Hand conditioning is a deliberate process of desensitizing and callusing the hands so that hard surfaces can be struck without feeling pain. I have personally observed a demonstration of hand conditioning so extreme that the individual could drive a nail into wood with his bare knuckle. For that trick, more than conditioning is needed; it takes endless hours of practice to develop the necessary technique.

There is absolutely no reason why the modern student of kung fu should condition his hands. You can enjoy all the benefits of kung fu practice without hardening and deforming your hands. There are potent social and medical arguments against hand conditioning.

For practice of the kung fu forms and routines, for fitness, recreation and physical development, hand conditioning is neither necessary nor appropriate.

For any kind of street defense, conditioned hands are a detriment, rather than an asset. In my view, the advocacy of hand conditioning today indicates an unreal, archaic attitude toward the world. In feudal times, when kung fu was developing, if an individual was wronged, or thought he was wronged, he took personal vengeance. By decent standards today, personal revenge is immoral; it is illegal, as well. Self-defense, in a society which regards itself as civilized, is defined as self-protection, not as punishment. It is against the law, and rightly so, to retaliate with greater force than is necessary for defense. There is no difference between defense and offense if the "defense" is vicious. A person who has heavily conditioned his hands appears to be an aggressor, whether or not he has started a fight. The burden of proof of self-defense is shifted onto the person who has conditioned his hands.

Heavy hand conditioning can affect manual dexterity—seriously and permanently. Aside from the loss of ability to use your hands for delicate or skillful work, the appearance of heavily conditioned hands is ugly. The youngster who enjoys showing off his "iron hands" while he is a teen-ager, could grow to regret them for the rest of his life!

It is a very risky sort of play-acting to imagine one's self a kung fu killer with iron hands and a heart to match.

WHAT IS THE POISON HAND?

Whereas the iron hand is a dramatic reference to hit with more-than-ordinary power, the "poison" hand is a highly dramatic reference to the skill of hitting at vulnerable body areas. Often, the two skills are confused and the body target area is said to be vulnerable when, in fact, it is the force of the blow which is the critical factor. An instance is the temple area. Striking at the temple is sometimes taught as a poison hand blow; the accurate blow is said to inflict severe damage. In point of fact, the area surrounding the eye is heavily protected by bone. As the ancients did *not* know, it is the *force* of a blow to the head which causes damage, not the accuracy. Hitting at the head with force, using any type of blow and hitting it at any angle which causes referral shock at the opposite part of the skull, can be a fatal blow.

The soft-style kung fu systems emphasize the really vulnerable body areas for clawing and stabbing hand blows. There is a great deal of emphasis on stabbing into the eyes and kicking into the groin, two tactics well-known to street-fighters, and in general, more appropriate for vicious attack than they are for self-defense.

It is not surprising that the knowledge of striking into vulnerable body areas has given rise to myths and fantasies which surround kung fu. I cannot here take the space to refute the many tall tales which are circulated about the amazing, secret knowledge that the old kung fu "masters" had. It is impossible, it seems, to find any real kung fu master who can repeat the incredible, fantastic, poison hand tricks we are told about, but the stories circulate, just the same. The observable "secret" tricks turn out to be the result, not of secret knowledge, but of years of diligent practice and training.

The tall tales of the kung fu master who could merely press at secret parts of the body, might possibly relate to pressing against the windpipe—no secret to hundreds of thousands of men who have had combat training. Any other pressure at the body would have to be fairly strong pressure to be effective.

There is entertainment value, but hardly any other kind of value to the stories of the kung fu masters whose poison hands could strike at secret parts of the body and cause *deferred* injury. There is no way to prove that story wrong, so it is repeated to delight our sense of the fantastic.

There is even a claim made for long-gone kung fu masters whose poison hands were more deadly at certain, secret hours of the day. My view is, of course a biased one. My bias is for physical education as against mystical thrills. I can participate, with pleasure, in super-men exploits, so long as a corner of my mind remembers that we are enchanted with them as entertainment. I am wild about John Henry and Paul Bunyan and the kung fu master who can do what no man could ever do—but I can be wild about then without having to believe that they are real! What would a person do, anyway, I wonder, if he learned the secret of the right time of day to use his poison hand? It could only be used aggressively for a planned attack; one could hardly ask that an assailant should make his attack during the favorable hours for defense.

FIGHT SCENES IN MOVIES

Many, many readers write to ask about a fight scene they have seen on television or in a movie. The question they ask is: "What was the wonderful style of fighting I saw on that program? It must really be good because the hero beat all those bigger guys with it."

It is very difficult for people to accept the fact that fight scenes on tv and in the movies are not real. We all recognize that those are not real doctors performing the operations in the tv medical series, we all know that cops and robbers are played by actors, not real policemen or real thieves — but fight scenes come across with enough realism to confuse the viewers. Fight scenes in movies are no more real than love scenes.

Movies and television stories follow a script. All the scenes are rehearsed over and over and they do not deviate from the script. The film shows are cast without regard for the actors' abilities as fighters or lovers; the actors are selected for their ability to act. The script decides, not the actor, who shall win and who shall lose the girl or the fight.

You must not confuse what happens on the screen with what is true, practical or realistic. When the actor who plays in a fight scene is known to have real ability as a fighter, it is more difficult to separate his real self from his screen image. But you must do that; to do otherwise is to be very innocent or very confused.

The bad guys lose the fight *not* because a superior form of fighting is used against them, but because the script decides when they lose. When I lived in Hollywood and operated a school there, I was often called upon to do work for the films. During those years I met many stunt men. Stunt men have very highly developed physical skills; they usually have much more fighting ability than the actors who play hero roles. These stunt men are cast as villains (who lose fights) because they can act the part well.

I have many times worked on a film in a triple capacity—fight-scene designer, trainer, villain. As the designer of the fight scene, I worked out every move of the fight for maximum excitement and action (not for practicality). As the trainer, I taught the film hero the techniques he would use in the fight scene. As the villain, I acted the part of the man who "lost" the fight to the hero whom I had trained to "win". All make-believe!

Television and movie scenes of fighting are for diversion, not instruction.

THE HORSE STANCE

Many readers have expressed curiosity about the horse stance in kung fu. It is characteristic of kung fu to begin practice techniques from the horse stance, or a variation of the basic horse stance and this has led to the assumption that there is an advantage inherent in the stance itself. In my view, this is not true.

Any fighting is done better from a strong, well-balanced stance which permits light and quick body movement. Most forms of sport fighting incorporate stances in training and in matches. The boxer's stance is a good example of a stance which gives stability and flexibility.

For self-defense, a stance is not necessarily efficient. A fast surprise attack doesn't allow time for taking a fancy stance. Against an assailant from the rear, a fighting stance is an obvious impossibility.

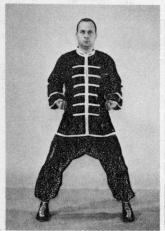 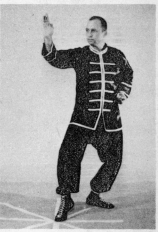

a.   b.

a. The basic horse stance, shown here, is a strong, solidly-balanced, stance; from the side it is also a well-guarded stance. It has the drawback of limiting free and light movement.

b. The cat stance is at the other end of the scale — it is a light, graceful, ready-to-move stance.

These are the two stances characteristic of kung fu practice routines. Attempts to justify the stances in terms of self-defense are not valid.

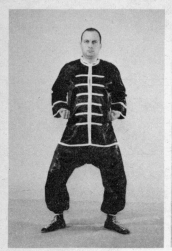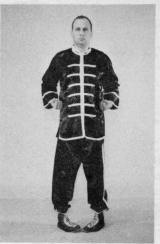

c.   d.

There are many variations of the basic horse stance,
some of them slight, stylistic nuances, such as the
position of the feet, as in c., and some of them are
extreme departures from the basic stance, for
example, the pigeon-toed posture in d., which is also
called a horse stance.

The horse stance is also used in some systems of kung
fu as "discipline" practice. The stance is held for
many minutes, which is difficult; or, it is held for
hours, which is extremely difficult. Holding an
immobile stance has no positive value—rather, the
opposite. Holding an immobile stance for long
periods of time bears no relation to development of
technique or tactics or physical fitness. Holding an
immobile stance for hours to "prove" oneself to a
"master" is an archaic, pointless exercise in ser-
vility. It is not discipline, it is obedience. There is no
need to accept feudal warrior training practices in
order to get the benefit of kung fu.

WILL THE REAL KUNG FU . . . ?

"How can I tell if the teacher is teaching an authentic style of kung fu?" asks the reader, or, he may ask the question: "What is the best style of karate, kung fu or some other system?"

My view is that *no specialty* of fighting, Oriental or European, is suitable for practical self-defense for the average person *in its ancient form*. My view is that *any* specialty of fighting is suitable for self-defense if the individual achieves *expert* skill in that method. Boxing, which is patently unsuitable for the average person with little skill, becomes a "deadly" art given the factors of physique, training, practice. It is hardly ever claimed that the average person can achieve the level of skill of a Sugar Ray Robinson by merely learning a few "tricks" of boxing. If a student with six months of training in kung fu routines thinks he is ready to defend himself against an experienced boxer, he is kidding himself, or he has been misled.

As I do not view kung fu as practical self-defense for most people, but rather a wonderful form of exercise, it is irrelevant to compare the merits of one style against the merits of another. Every teacher of every system of karate, kung fu or any other system, makes the claim that his system is the best, the only authentic, the only true, the only legitimate, style of karate. Even within the same system of kung fu, there is a clash of opinion as to which sub-style is best. The reason that teachers of each system claim to be the best, is that each one is making a personal judgement. If the teachers of kenpo karate and the teachers of kung fu karate and the teachers of

Okinawa-te, and so on, continue to prefer their own styles, it is apparent that in all these years they have not succeeded in convincing *each other* of any inherent superiority of method. The choice, for the student, then, has to be based on the same thing—personal preference.

The best style or system of karate is the one which appeals to you.

But, persists, the questioner, if kung fu is older than the other Oriental systems of karate, doesn't that mean that it is more authentic? Nothing is better merely because it is an old or a new procedure. Burning and drowning witches is an authentically ancient practice and napalming people is a new one. Procedures and practices must be evaluated on their worth, not on their age. It was once the authentic practice to perform surgery without anesthetics; would you choose the old method because it is old, or would you prefer the new, painless method? The original style of boxing included the practice of wearing spiked gloves; the winner killed the loser. Can you conceive of anyone suggesting that we return to the authentic, original form of boxing?

MISCELLANY

ARE THERE BELTS & DEGREES IN KUNG FU? Until fairly recently, it has been the custom in most systems of kung fu *not* to grade achievement or progress by awarding colored belts to indicate rank. There seems to be a change in the policy developing now, and it appears that the trend is toward an increase in recognition of proficiency through colored belts, patches, certificates and other rank indicators.

DOES KUNG FU HAVE TOURNAMENT? Most systems of kung fu do not have contest or engage in sports tournament. There have been individuals trained in kung fu who have entered karate contest. There, they performed with varying degrees of success, according to individual skill. Competition in karate has consistently indicated that it is not the *style* that wins, but the individual's level of skill.

DOES KUNG FU TRAINING INCLUDE WEAPONS? Some systems of kung fu teach weapons practice routines, that is, routines in which weapons are simulated. It is highly unlikely that the original kung fu included weapons, but that swords, spears, knives, axes, truncheons, tridents, etc, were included as later developments.

In conclusion, let me thank you for your many letters and your expressions of interest and enthusiasm. Although I cannot make separate replies, I read your letters carefully, with pleasure and gratitude.

Sincerely yours,

Bruce Tegner

PRACTICE PROCEDURES

HOW LONG TO PRACTICE. Practice time will vary greatly from one person to another. The factors which will determine the correct amount of time for you are: available time, physical condition and the degree of interest. One individual might spend an agreeable and profitable ten minutes a day practicing kung fu or tai chi, while another might spend an hour or more.

MENTAL PRACTICE. Scientific study and experiments have revealed an interesting correlation between physical practice and mental rehearsal of the physical skill which has been learned through physical performance. After the movements of kung fu and tai chi have been learned, you can enhance the ability to perform them through mental review. By thinking about them, by visualizing them, by rehearsing them in sequence, mentally, you can retain and improve your skill. This kind of mental drill is not a mystical or mysterious process, it is a straightforward learning process.

DIRECTION REFERENCES. When the instructions are given in compass points, it is easier to follow them if you face the actual point of reference. When the directions are given as "front, rear, right and left" they are to be read as follows:

FRONT always means the direction you face as you begin a sequence. RIGHT and LEFT are stationary points, and are always left or right of the FRONT starting position. REAR is a stationary point behind the FRONT starting position.

FORWARD and BACKWARD are not fixed points; they refer to movement forward or back from the direction you face when the instruction is given.

MEMORIZING THE ROUTINES

A major benefit to be had from practicing kung fu and tai chi is the mental stimulation/relaxation which comes from concentrating on learning the routines. The duality of stimulation/relaxation through concentration is not unique to kung fu or tai chi, but kung fu and tai chi are remarkably effective for the purpose. As in many other activities which require alert attention, you will gain benefits in proportion to your involvement; the more you give to kung fu and tai chi, the more you will benefit.

Mental stimulation results from the amount of mental effort required to comprehend and memorize the movements and sequences of movements. Relaxation results from diverting your thoughts away from the worrisome daily preoccupations and minor frustrations of life and fixing them on a fresh and absorbing activity for mind and body.

There are two distinct ways of memorizing the material. Choose the one which suits your temperament and your situation.

THE SHORT-GROUP METHOD. This method of learning is excellent for those whose practice time at any one session is limited and for those who are engaging in solo practice without anyone to help them. Because a person practicing altogether alone must refer to the book at frequent intervals to learn the movements, the short-group method is appropriate.

As the name implies, the short-group method involves taking small parts of each routine, from four to six movements, and practicing that small portion over and over. When that small sequence is learned, you proceed to learn the next few movements and practice those intensively.

When you have practiced five or six short groups, you assemble them into one, longer sequence. Then you begin the next short groups. When you have learned the next five or six groups, assemble them into one sequence and then join the two longer sequences into one.

Proceed in this manner until you have learned all the movements of a routine and can perform them in a single, uninterrupted sequence.

THE LONG-GROUP METHOD. If you have a practice partner who can read the movements aloud as you perform them, or if you find this method more to your liking, follow this procedure: practice the maximum number of movements of a routine which you can cover in a single session.

When the long-group method is used, progress in memorization does not appear to be as rapid as when the short-group method is used, but, for many individuals, the long-group method is suitable. If you are not sure which of the two methods is better for you, try them both and select the one which gives *you* the best results.

Specialists in the psychology of learning and memory believe that the long-group method of memorizing results in longer retention of the learned material. Using the long-group method, you will not memorize the movements in sequence as quickly as in the short-group method, but it is likely that you will remember them better and for a longer time once you do memorize them.

If you do not have a practice partner, you might find someone who would be willing to read the movements aloud to you so that you can practice without constant references to the book, though you should study the photos carefully before you begin, so that you will have a clear mental image of the gesture of each movement.

Solo practice or group practice will yield benefits of a somewhat different character. For those of you who have no choice except to practice alone, or for those of you who prefer to practice alone, there is the benefit of complete absorption in the performance of the movements without the distraction of company. Whether you engage in solo practice through choice or through necessity, make the most of it.

For those individuals who enjoy and prefer group activity, and have the opportunity to work with a group, kung fu and tai chi practice with partners is an excellent mode of practice. If you have one person who will join you in practicing the movements, you can help each other, read aloud to each other and do the two-man forms together.

If you have the time and inclination, you could even organize a group to practice together for recreation. It is not necessary for any of you to have had previous experience to make this an enjoyable and worthwhile activity. In a group, each person takes a turn reading the instructions to the group.

Whether you practice alone or with a group, whether you use the short-group method or the long-group method, you will refer to the photos less and less as you progress. Finally, you should arrive at a stage where you can perform the routines purely from memory; you will use the book as a reference and for refresher practice.

KUNG FU

STANCES IN THE FORMS

1. BASIC HORSE STANCE. This is the basic stance, facing front. This stance was originally called the horse-riding stance, which gives a good notion of the basic gesture. Imagine that you are on horseback: knees are bent, feet point straight ahead, back is erect and fists are held at sides.

2. The horse stance is also used facing to the side, as in this photo.

3. CAT STANCE. This is characteristic of kung fu practice routines, shown here with a slashing hand position. Weight is almost entirely placed on the rear leg and the rear foot is at an angle, as shown. The forward foot bears very little weight on the ball. In contrast to the horse stance, which is a strong, heavy, stance, the cat stance is a light, ready-for-movement posture.

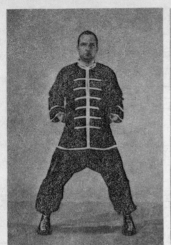

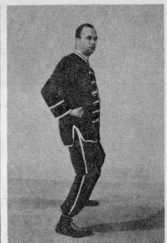

1

2

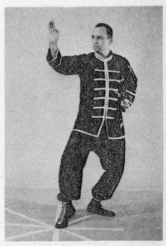

3

MODES OF MOVING

There are stylized modes of moving in kung fu which are utilized in the practice routines. As is true of the hand blows, some of these moving procedures are practical, while some of them have no practical application in the sense that they might be of value in a defense situation on the street. Those which do not have a modern defense application are, nevertheless, necessary to learn if you wish to perform the kung fu routines and they have the value of body-movement exercise.

The instructions for modes of moving are given in compass points and it will be easier for you to follow them if you move toward the actual compass point as your directional reference.

4. STEPPING HORSE. Begin from the basic horse stance, facing forward toward the east.

5. Turning clockwise, step around (forward) with your left foot to face south.

6. Turning clockwise, step around (back) with your right foot to face west.

7. Turning clockwise, step around (forward) with your left foot to face north. Turning clockwise, step around (back) with your right foot to face the starting position, east, as in photo 4.

Another mode of practicing the moving horse stance is to keep one foot in place, to pivot on that foot and turn in the four directions by moving the other foot four steps clockwise or four steps counterclockwise. This is practiced alternating the foot which is the pivot point.

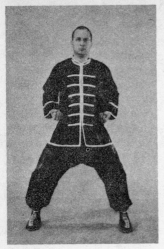

4

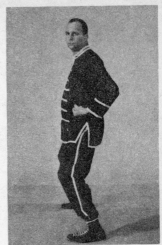

5

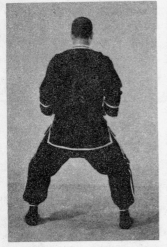

6

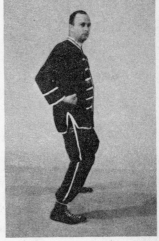

7

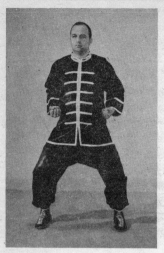 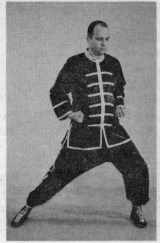

8   9

8. SIDE STEPPING. Begin from the standard horse stance.

9. Keeping your left foot in place, take a wide step to the side with your right foot. Then slide the left foot into place so that you are in the starting position in photo 8. Body balance is maintained through the shift from position to position. The step is practiced from one side to the other.

10. The following is a two-step move. From the basic horse stance, take a medium step to the right with your right foot.

11. Draw your left foot up to the right foot. Without hesitation, take another step with your right foot to return to the original horse stance position.

This mode of moving lets you cover more distance, but puts you in a very awkward, vulnerable position during the instant when your feet are together.

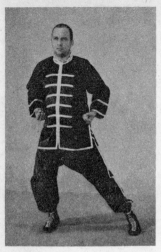

10

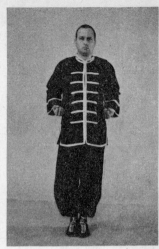

11

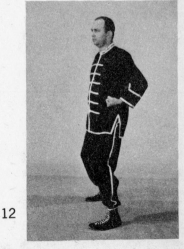

12

12. CROSS-OVER STEP. Start in the basic horse stance; shift your weight onto your left foot.

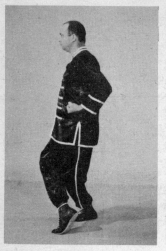 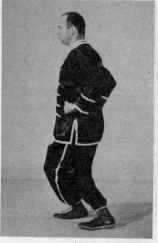

13   14

13. Lightly cross your right foot over your left, keeping your body weight over your center of gravity to minimize the danger of loss of balance. Place your weight onto your right foot and then step out with your left foot so that you are in the starting horse stance.

14. The other mode of cross-stepping is done by taking the first step behind, rather than in front of the stationary foot. From the starting horse stance, take a step behind your left foot with your right foot. As you transfer body weight to your right foot, step out with your left foot to put you into the starting horse stance.

Emphasis on the cross-over step is characteristic of kung fu; most other systems of karate and related styles of fighting expressly warn against this style of moving because it places the body in very awkward, vulnerable position. It occurs in kung fu forms and is practiced for performance of those forms.

CIRCLE STEP. The forward, circular-step mode of moving is characteristic of kung fu and is also practiced in other styles of karate.

Ground contact is maintained as you move; the center of gravity is well under your body. There is a feeling of strong balance maintained throughout the movements, and the gesture is graceful.

There is no hesitation between the movements; they flow together.

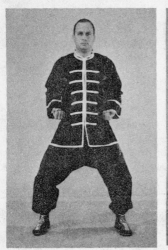   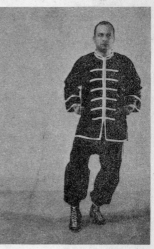

15   16

15. Begin from horse stance.

16. As weight is shifted to the left foot, the right foot is drawn toward the left foot in a circular motion.

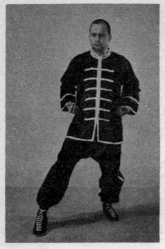 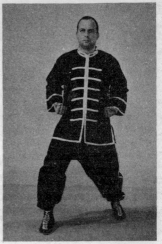

17   18

17. The circular motion continues and the right foot is advanced as shown.

18. After the right foot reaches its farthest extension in the step, weight is transferred to that foot and the process is repeated, this time with the left foot.

This manner of moving is practiced forward and to the rear. The gliding, rounded movement of this way of changing position resembles skating.

HAND BLOWS

Most of the hand blows which are used in kung fu are indistinguishable from the hand blows of other styles of karate.

Kung fu styles vary—some preferring the power punching blows and others preferring the clawing, poking finger stabs which rely on speed.

The clawing and stabbing hand blows are common in kung fu practice routines and will be illustrated in the forms.

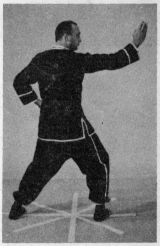

19

19. KNIFE-SLASH BLOW. The most common karate hand blow, using the edge of the open hand. This hand blow is found in all styles of karate, as well as in jiu jitsu and related styles of weaponless fighting. It is known by many different names—the sword hand, the knife blade, the judo chop, the thousand hand blow, and more. No matter what name is used to describe it, it is the same blow.

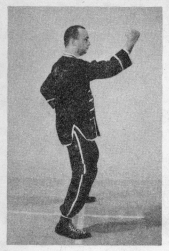 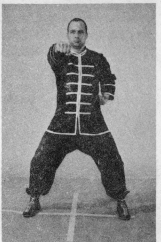

20   21

When the hand is held as in photo 19, but the tips of the fingers are used for poking, thrusting blows, it is called the KNIFE-POINT BLOW.

20. HAMMER BLOW. This is another common karate blow, found in many different styles of karate. The action resembles the action of a hammer, properly used; the recoil, bounce-back effect should be obvious.

21. RAM'S HEAD BLOW. A power blow; the striking area is at the two large knuckles. Used with palm down, as shown, or with palm inward or upward.

22. DOUBLE RAM'S HEAD BLOW.

23. SCORPION BLOW. Back knuckle blow with circular, sweeping action preceding delivery. This is not a power blow, but has speed and whip.

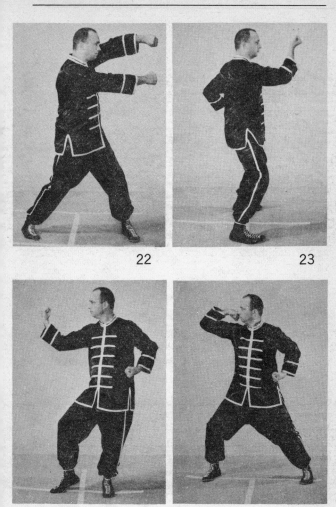

22

23

24

25

24. POUNDING WAVE BLOW. This blow is delivered with dramatic crashing gesture.

25. MONKEY BLOW. Elbow blow; striking with flat area just above or below the point of the elbow.

26. ROCK SMASH BLOW. Heel-of-the-palm blow.

27. TIGER CLAW. Characteristic of kung fu preference for clawing hand blows. In this version, all
the fingers are used. Other variations utilize bunched
fingers or one, two or three fingers used for a stabbing action.

KICKING

The basic kicking techniques of kung fu are similar
to those of other styles of karate, though in the practice routines they seem different because of the
stylistic manner of performance. The hard styles of
kung fu emphasize kicking practice more than the
soft styles do.

In the practice forms which follow, the kicks which
occur most frequently are the lightning kick and the
dragon stamp. These are shown here; other kicks
will be taught the first time they occur in a routine.

28. LIGHTNING KICK. A fast, snappy kick using
the bottom or side of the shoe as the striking point.
Speed is the essential factor in the delivery of this
technique.

29. DRAGON STAMP. This is a power kick
delivered with the bottom of the shoe. The gesture of
the kick clearly indicates strength, rather than speed.

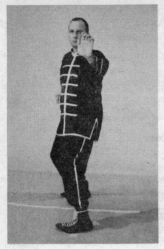
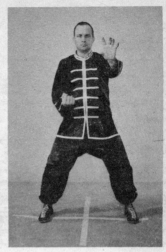

26   27

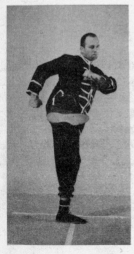
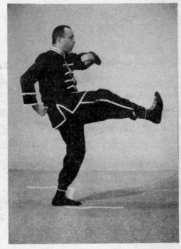

28   29

APPLICATION OF HAND BLOWS

Characteristic of kung fu is the gesture of follow-through in the application of hand blows. The principle of action-reaction is used more than the single-blow tactic.

The man at the left is shown as a reference point.

30-31. From a high, raised position, right man delivers a hammer blow.

32. His striking hand follows through completely, putting body power behind the blow and winding up for the reaction blow.

33. The reaction blow is a pounding wave, which would be carried through fully to the other side, preparing for another counteraction blow.

The principle works whether it is one hand or both hands delivering blows; there is the constant, moving action from one blow to the next. The more sophisticated the student is in his development, the more he will be able to carry on the action from blow to blow in the appropriate manner.

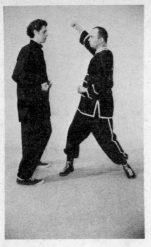

30

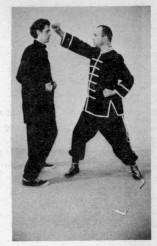

31

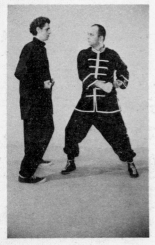

32

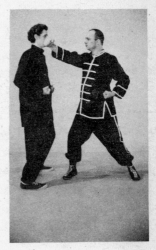

33

BLOCKS & PARRIES

34. WHIPPING BRANCH (High Slashing Block). To block an attack from high, left, left man uses the whipping branch to deflect the blow. The action of the block is like that which results when a branch is pulled as far as possible and suddenly released.

The direction of the block is upward and outward and the hand can be held open or fisted. The striking point is the forearm; the block is applied with either arm.

35. A variation of the whipping branch is this block/parry with the forearm. Although the whipping action is present, there is greater power in the block.

36. It can be applied with the inside or outside of the forearm, cross-body or back-handed, as shown.

37. LEAPING DEER (Rising Forearm Block). The action of this block is an abrupt, springing up, as though to stop and deflect a high blow coming directly forward.

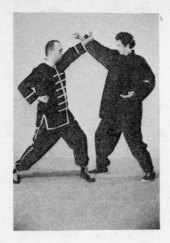

34

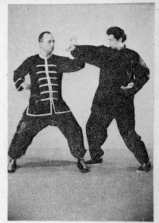

35

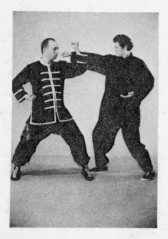

36

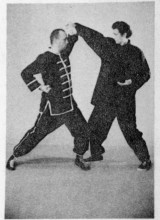

37

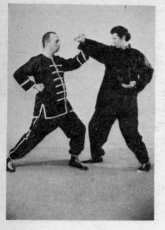

38

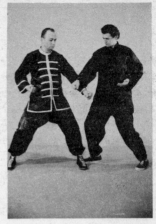

39

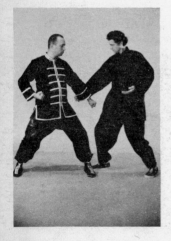

40

38. ROCK SMASH (Heel-of-Palm Parry). The rock smash, heel-of-palm, parry is used against a cross-body blow and it fully deflects the intended blow. In the form, the rock smash can be practiced with contact, since it is not a blow, but a parry.

39. BOULDER BLOCK (Forearm Block). The boulder block counters the intended blow with greater force than the whipping branch. In the forms, the boulder block is practiced to simulate powerful, crashing action.

40. The boulder block is also practiced back-handed, as in this photo.

SWOOPING BIRD PARRY. In contrast to the forearm block, which is a hard-style method of blocking, there is the swooping bird parry, characteristic of soft-style kung fu and also used in aikido practice forms.

The hard-style methods are dynamic and opposi-tional; they are practiced with gestures which simulate full strength and power.

The soft actions are based on the principle of "going with" the blow, rather than opposing it with greater force. "Going with" implies the utilization of the opponent's energy. In the swooping actions the blows are deflected, not opposed.

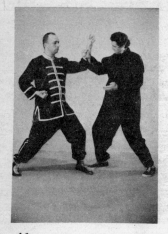

41

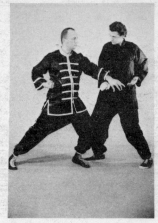

42

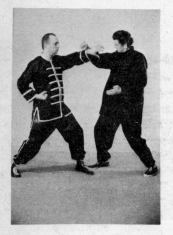

43

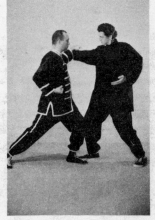

44

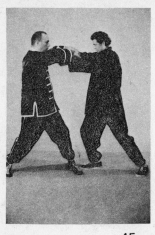 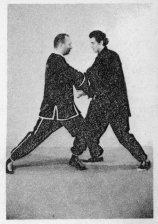

45   46

41. As right man punches, left man begins his circular, swooping action. . . .

42. . . . and deflects the blow. The hand may be held open, claw-like as shown in the photos, or it may be fisted. The action is flowing and circular.

43-44. A similar action, but outward, is shown here to deflect right man's intended punch. The full, circular action, carried through properly, places your forearm onto his forearm as his arm is moved downward.

45-46. The double-handed swooping parry is used against two-handed punches. This technique does not relate very much to what might be called practical situations, but as a coordination exercise it is excellent, and it is necessary to learn in order to perform the kung fu forms in which it appears.

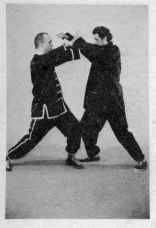 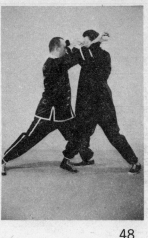

47   48

As the double punch approaches, both arms swoop
outward to parry in a circular movement. The contact
with his arms is made from the top so that your right
hand makes a clockwise circle as your left hand
makes a counterclockwise circle.

47. This is the same action, reversed.

48. The swooping circle made by the right hand is
counterclockwise; the left hand makes a clockwise
circle.

DODGING & DUCKING

49. DODGING/BLOCK. The essential action of this method of evading the attack is a simultaneous movement of the body as the arm is raised to block. Because the block is used, it is only necessary to move the body slightly out of range of the oncoming attack.

I would like to repeat here, for emphasis, comments made earlier in the book with respect to traditional procedures as contrasted with practical procedures.

Verified by experience, is the fact that a student with relatively little training and only a functional level of skill can use the blocking method shown in photo 49. That is, he can use it for practical self-defense in addition to using it as a formal technique in a practice routine.

49

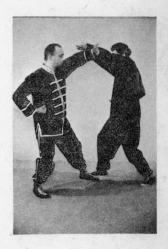

In contrast, the ducking and blocking procedure shown in photos 50 and 51 can only be used if the student has had a great deal of practice and training and has achieved a high level of skill which he maintains through constant practice. This technique occurs in kung fu forms, but only the exceptional person could use it effectively for street defense. As exercise it is excellent and if you wish to practice the kung fu forms, you will learn the traditional as well as the practical procedures.

50. LOW DODGE & COUNTER. In this procedure the dodge and counterblow are not simultaneous, but are two distinct actions. The first action is a very low dodge, to the side.

51. The second action is a hand blow.

52. LOW DUCK & BLOCK. The duck and block actions are simultaneous. As the attack is made, left man squats and blocks upward.

53. LOW SQUAT & HIT. This procedure is two separate actions. The first action is a very low squat as the attack is made.

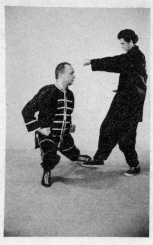

50

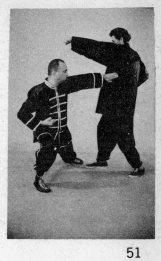

51

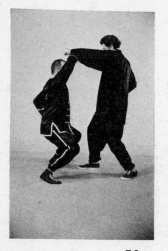

52

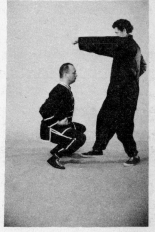

53

54. The second action is
a counterblow into the
midsection.

The comments which I
have made with respect
to the technique in pho-
tos 50 and 51, apply
equally to the technique
above.

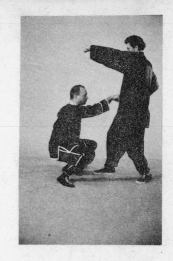

54

SALUTATION

These are the ceremonial movements which precede
each single-man form. The symbolism of these
movements may not have any meaning to the
Western student. They are the stylized, classical
manner of beginning the forms. Different schools
of kung fu have ritualized the salutation in different
movements. In general, they indicate respect for the
teacher, hidden strength, humility, prayer and
alertness.

This salutation series is a typical kung fu procedure.

The five movements of salutation: These are done
slowly, with hesitation between the movements.

55. The awareness position or, the position of
attention: Feet together, hands at sides; straight
but relaxed body.

56. Hidden strength position: The right fist is
brought back to the left hip and covered by the left
hand, palm down.

57. Position of humility: Take a step back with the right foot and go down on the right knee as the covered fist is brought to the right hip.

58. Reverent position: As you rise from position of humility, pivot on left foot and stand facing right. The covered fist is raised, palm out.

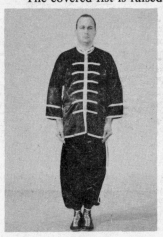

55

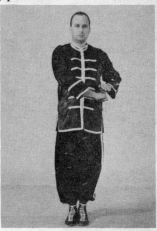

56

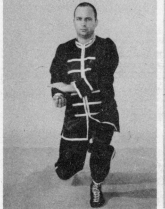

57

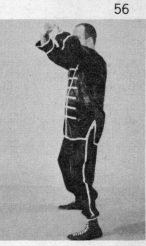

58

59. Position of alertness: Take a step counterclockwise with your left foot into horse stance facing front; your right fist is held chin high.

60. By bringing both fists to hips, palm up, you assume the standard horse stance, which is, properly speaking, the first movement of each form.

STRAIGHT LINE FORM

A basic form for the beginner, this six-movement form utilizes a few simple hand blows. The purpose of practicing this form is to let you become accustomed to combining several movements in characteristic kung fu manner.

The move from action to action is flowing and continuous, with exaggerated, stylized gestures.

You can draw a line, or imagine one; all the action moves back and forth along this line.

Start in the position of attention.

61. Move slowly into the horse stance, with your arms making circular, flowing movements into the fist-up position.

62. Pivot on the balls of both feet, turning your upper body toward the left as you deliver left boulder block downward; your right fist stays in place.

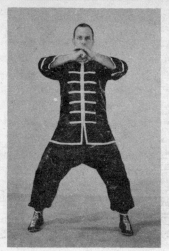

59

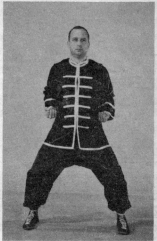

60

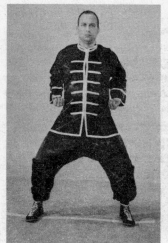

61

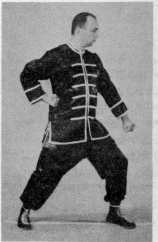

62

63. Turning your body counterclockwise, assume a horse stance on the line, facing rear; as you turn, deliver tiger-claw thrust with your right hand as you draw your left fist to your left hip.

64. Turning clockwise, swing your body around to assume a horse stance on the line, facing forward. As you turn, deliver right, outward, whipping branch blow as your left fist is brought to your left hip.

The gesture of the eagle-beak blow is made by bunching the fingers together and making snappy, pecking motions, forward.

65. Turning clockwise, turn to face the rear; as you turn, deliver a left eagle-beak blow as your right fist is brought to your right hip.

66. Turning counterclockwise, return to the starting horse stance on the line, facing front. Return to a position of attention.

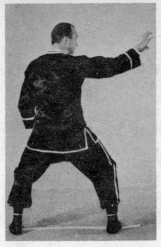
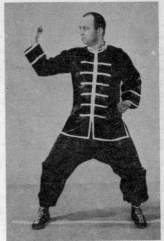

63

64

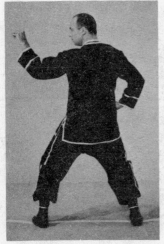
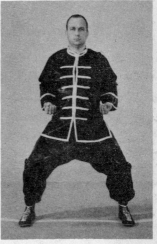

65

66

ZIG-ZAG LINE FORM

Start from the position of attention.

67. Assume the horse stance, facing front.

68. Right foot and right fist kept in place, take a short step left with your left foot as you deliver an outward whipping-branch blow with your left arm.

69. Turning counterclockwise, pivot on your left foot, swing body around to face rear; as you turn, bring left fist to hip, deliver knife-slash blow with right hand.

70. Turning clockwise, pivot on left foot so that your body faces left; look front and deliver outward whipping-branch block with right arm; left fist is brought to hip.

71. Turning clockwise, pivot on right foot and swing body around until you face right; look front, deliver hammer blow with left fist as your right fist is brought to hip.

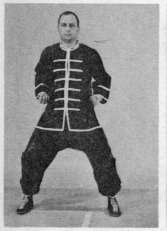
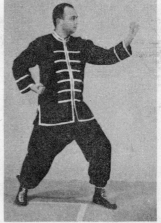

67   68

72. Turning counterclockwise, pivot on right foot, taking step back with left foot to assume horse stance facing front but looking left; as you turn, bring right fist to hip, deliver boulder block downward with left arm.

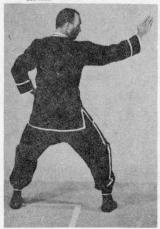

69

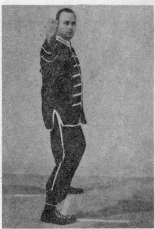

70

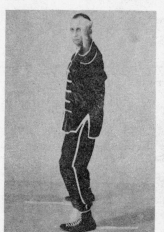

71

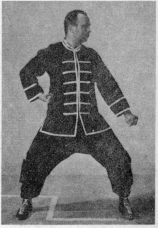

72

73. Pivot on left foot, turning counterclockwise to face left and deliver forward dragon stamp with right foot; as you kick, your left forearm is raised, as shown.

74. Place your right foot down, your body faces left; look front as you deliver downward boulder block with right forearm, left fist at hip.

75. Turn clockwise, pivot around on right foot and deliver dragon stamp front with left foot as you deliver ram's-head punch with right fist.

Return to horse stance, facing front. Return to position of attention.

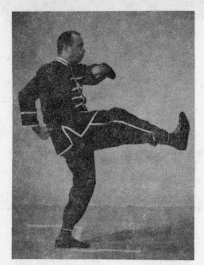

73

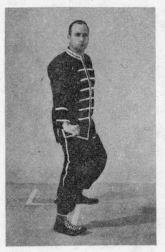

74

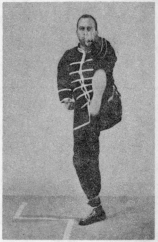

75

KUNG LINE FORM

Start from position of attention.

76. Assume horse stance.

77. Right foot and fist in place, take a short step to left side with left foot as you deliver leaping-deer block with left arm.

78. Pivot on left foot, swing your body counter-clockwise to face rear; as you bring your left fist to hip, deliver ram's-head punch with right fist.

79. Right foot in place, take short step to right with left foot and deliver downward boulder block with left arm as you bring right fist to hip.

80. Pivot on left foot, turning counterclockwise to face right and deliver dragon stamp with right foot, bringing both fists to hips.

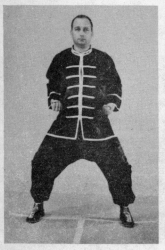
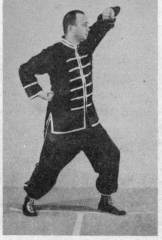

76   77

81. As kicking foot is placed down, pivot on left foot, turning counterclockwise to face front; right hand in place, deliver leaping-deer block upward with left arm.

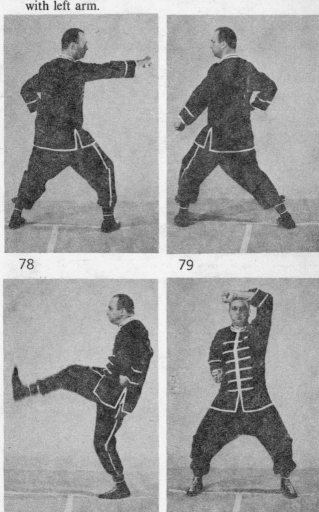

78

79

80

81

82. Take a step to the front with your right foot and pivot on the balls of both feet to face left as you deliver scorpion blow with right hand, left fist at hip.

83. Turning clockwise, pivot on right foot and swing your body around to face right; look front, deliver left boulder block downward, right fist to hip.

84. Pivot counterclockwise on left foot to make a half-circle; deliver lightning kick with right foot.

85. As kicking foot is placed down, deliver boulder block with right arm.

86. Step to right side with right foot, turning body clockwise to face front; deliver boulder block down with right arm, left fist at hip.

87. Pivot clockwise on right foot, deliver dragon stamp to right with left foot.

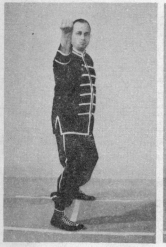
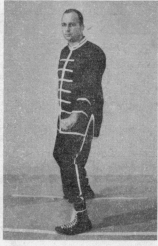

82   83

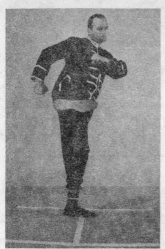

84

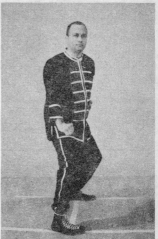

85

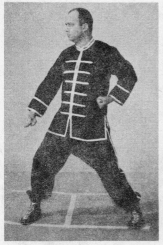

86

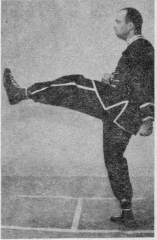

87

88. Place kicking foot down to face rear; deliver boulder block downward with right arm as you look left.

89. Turn clockwise, pivot on right foot, swing around so that your feet point front, but body is turned to left and you look left; deliver double ram's-head blows.

90. Swing body around counterclockwise, pivot on right foot, face rear; deliver tiger-claw blow to rear with left hand.

91. As you step to rear with right foot, deliver monkey blow with right elbow.

92. Turning clockwise, step around with left foot to face left; look to rear and deliver tiger-claw blow with left hand.

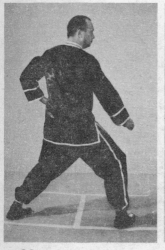

88

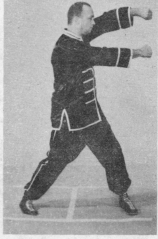

89

93. Turning counterclockwise, step around with right foot to face right; look to rear and deliver tiger-claw blow with right hand.

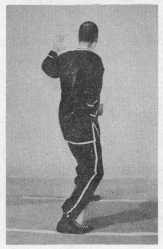

90

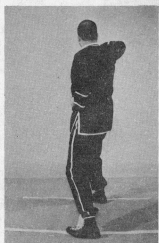

91

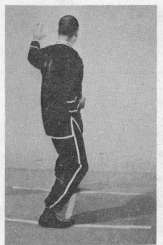

92

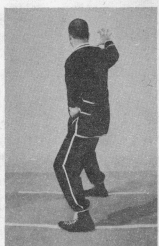

93

94. Pivot on right foot, swinging body clockwise to face rear, as you turn, deliver dragon stamp with left foot.

95. Place kicking foot down, feet point rear, body turned toward left; look left, deliver boulder block downward with right arm.

96. Pivot on right foot, swing body clockwise so that feet point front but body is turned left; look left and deliver tiger-claw blow with left hand.

97. Twist body to look right as you deliver whipping-branch block with right arm.

98. Pivot on right foot, swing body around to face rear; deliver monkey blow with left elbow.

99. No footwork; deliver boulder block down with left arm.

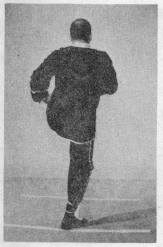

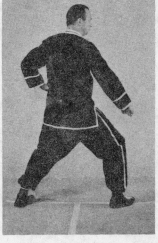

94   95

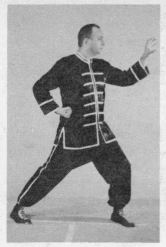

96

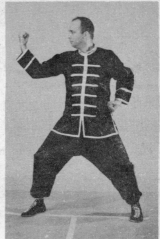

97

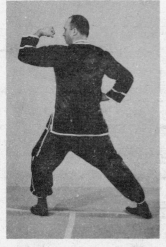

98

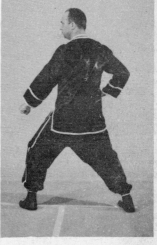

99

100. Swing body counter-
clockwise, pivot on right
foot, face front; look right,
deliver monkey blow to
right with right elbow.

Return to horse stance.
Return to position of
attention.

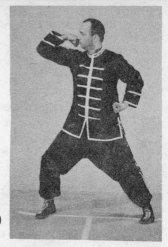

100

RICE LINE FORM

This is the traditional name given to a form which
moves around in a generally circular fashion, as
though on the spokes of a wheel, sometimes moving
from spoke to spoke around the rim and sometimes
moving through the hub. It is so called, not because
of any resemblance to the shape of a rice kernel,
but of a similarity to the written Chinese character
for rice.

Start from position of attention.

101. Assume horse stance.

102. Feet in place, shift body weight onto right foot,
drawing body to right; deliver slow, low, knife-slash
blow with left hand.

103. Pivot on left foot, swing body counterclockwise
to face rear, deliver knife-slash blow with right hand.

104. Pivot on left foot, swing body counterclockwise to face right in cat stance, with right foot forward; deliver knife-slash block upward with right hand.

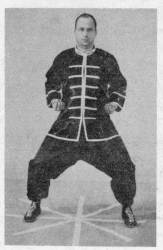

101

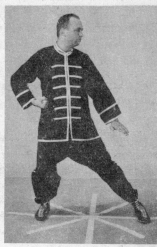

102

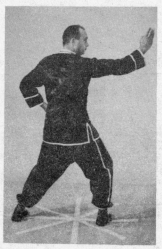

103

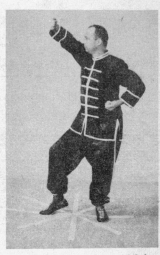

104

105. Turning clockwise, step with your left foot to face rear; look right and deliver knife-point blow with left hand.

106. Turning counterclockwise, step with your left foot so that your body faces right; look front, deliver knife-slash blow low with left hand.

107. Pivot on left foot to face front as you deliver dragon stamp with right foot, both fists at hips.

108. Place kicking foot down to face right front as you look right and deliver a whipping-branch block outward with right arm.

109. Moving clockwise, step around with left foot to face rear; look right and deliver monkey blow with left elbow.

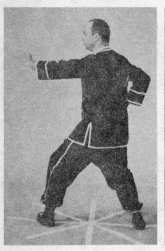 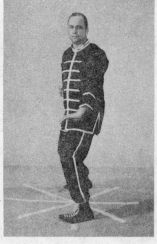

105   106

110. Back pivot counterclockwise, swinging around in a three-quarter circle to face left-rear; as you turn, deliver knife-slash blow outward with left hand.

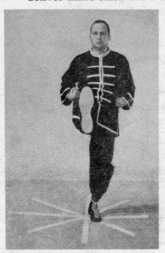

107

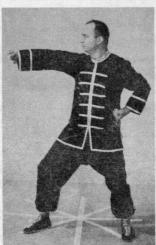

108

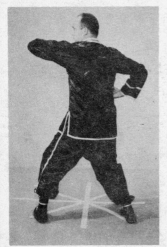

109

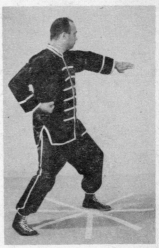

110

111. Moving counterclockwise, step to left-rear with right foot as you deliver ram's-head blow with right hand.

112. Take step to rear with right foot as you deliver leaping-deer block up, with right arm.

113. Pivot on right foot, take step with left foot moving clockwise to face left; look rear, deliver side hammer blow with left hand.

114. Back pivot, stepping clockwise with your right foot to face front; look left, deliver knife-slash blow with left hand.

115. Turning counterclockwise, step around with right foot to face rear; look left, deliver buffalo-horn blow with right hand. (Center knuckle punch.)

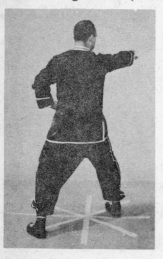

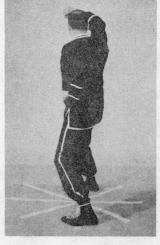

111   112

116. Moving clockwise, step around to right-front into a cat stance with right foot forward; right hand is raised into knife-slash position.

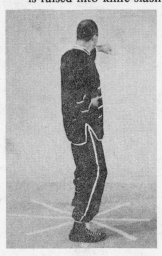

113

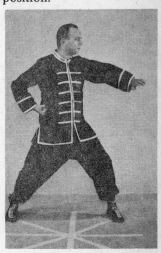

114

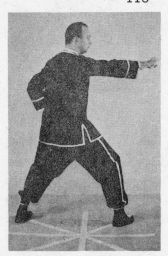

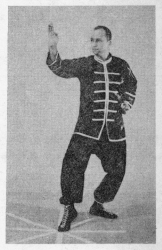

116

117. Step to right front with left foot; deliver tiger-claw blow with left hand.

118. Step back with right foot to face front in horse stance; both hands are in talon position; hands will make a circular reaching movement in the transition between this and the next action.

The talon position is not so much a hand blow position as it is a preliminary hand position for moving into clawing or stabbing actions.

119. Talon hands are extended fully forward and continue the circular action as you make the next movement.

120. Return to position of attention with fists at hips.

Return to position of attention.

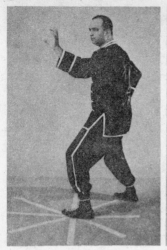

117

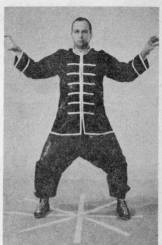

118

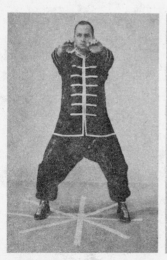

119

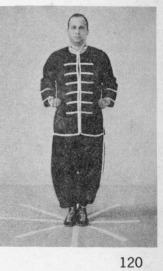

120

TWO-MAN FORM

The two-man forms of kung fu resemble the stylized two-man forms of other styles of karate, although this form has a longer sequence than is ordinarily found in karate forms.

The common manner of practicing two-man forms in most styles of karate is a series of actions of: attack, defense and counter-attack, after which the two men return to the starting position to begin another series. In this kung fu form, there is a sequence of attack, defense, counter-attack, defense, counter-counter-attack, and so on for a total of ten complete actions, in a smooth, continuous action.

Although most styles of kung fu do not include contest or tournament work, these forms resemble a give-and-take manner of practice, which is clearly the forerunner of sparring styles found in later types of karate.

This particular kung fu form has been selected for presentation because of the variety of blows and counter-blows it uses. It is representative of a form practiced by fairly advanced students.

Please note that, in practice, the intended attack is not permitted to be finished; the defense begins *as* the attacking blow is in progress. I have included photos of the *intended* attack to show exactly what is being defended against. The action of the form, in other words, goes from photo 122 to photo 124 *without* the intended attack carried through as in photo 123.

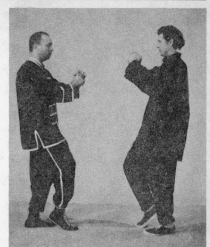

121

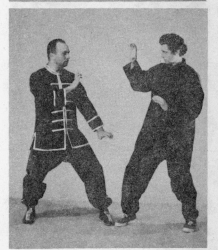

122

121. Salutation. This is the conventional beginning for the two-man forms. There is no bow as would be typical of other styles of karate.

122. Left man assumes side horse stance with low guard; right man assumes side horse stance with high guard.

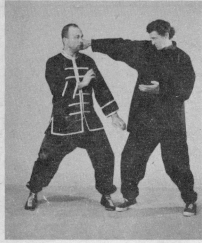

123

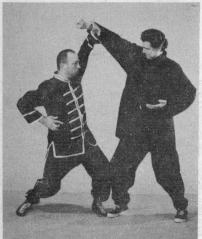

124

123. Right man intends attack with ram's-head blow toward head.

124. The attack is stopped by left man using leaping-deer block.

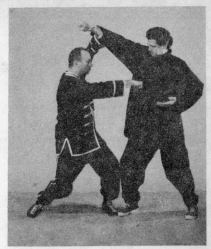

125

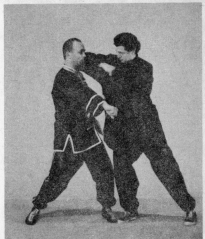

126

125. Left man intends ram's-head punch into mid-section.

126. Intended blow is stopped with low boulder block; right man counters with monkey blow with right elbow.

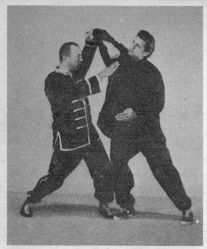

127

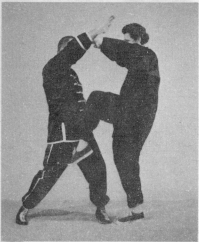

128

127. Intended monkey-blow counter is stopped by left man using leaping-deer block; he counters with knife-point blow with his right hand.

128. Right man stops intended knife-point blow using leaping-deer block with his left arm; he counters with raised-hoof kick, as shown in the photo.

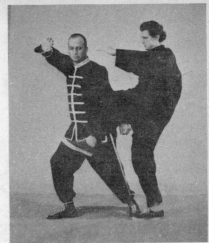

129

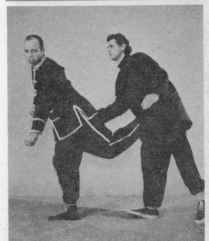

130

129. Intended kick is stopped with a low whipping-branch parry.

130. Left man counters with a horse kick—a backward stamp . . .

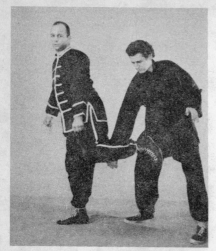

131

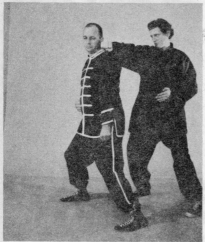

132

131. . . . which the right man parries, using the whipping branch.

132. Right man counters with side hammer blow.

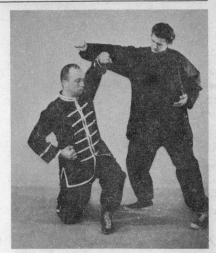

133

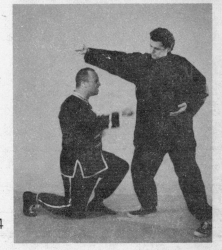

134

133. Left man drops to right knee as he stops intended hammer blow with leaping-deer block.

134. He pivots to face right man and counters with ram's-head punch.

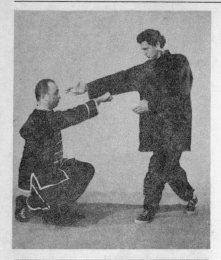

135

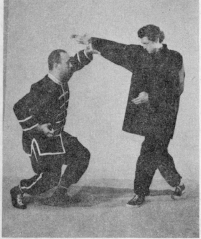

136

135. Right man evades intended blow by stepping back and counters with knife-point blow.

136. Left man rises to stop intended knife-point blow using whipping-branch block, palm up.

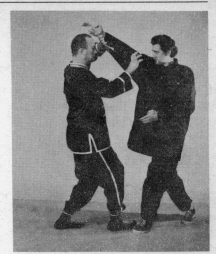

137

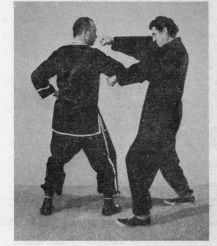

138

137. Left man counters with tiger-claw blow into face.

138. Right man stops intended tiger-claw blow by using whipping-branch parry; he counters with ram's-head punch.

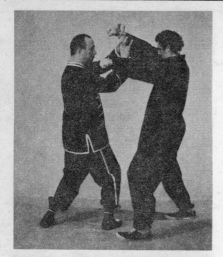

139

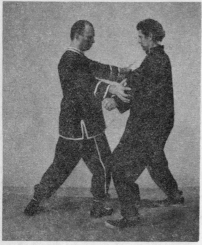

140

139-140. Left man stops intended ram's-head punch using swooping-bird parry.

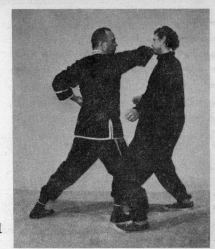

141

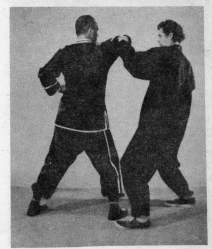

142

141. Left man intends monkey blow with right elbow.

142. Right man stops intended monkey blow using rock-smash parry with left hand.

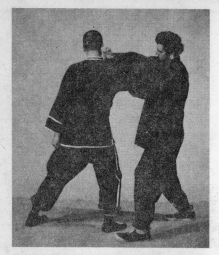

143

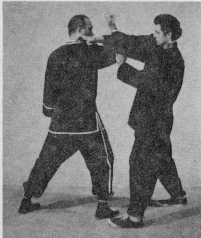

144

143. Right man counters with knife-slash blow into neck.

144. Left man stops intended blow with backhanded whipping-branch block.

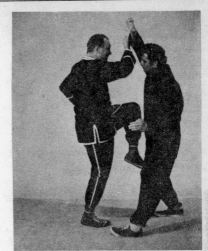

145

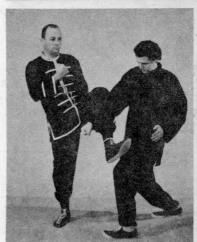

146

145. Left man counters with raised-hoof kick.

146. Right man stops intended kick with whipping-branch parry.

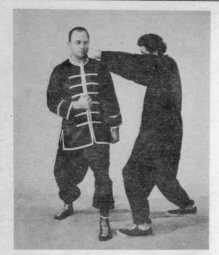

147

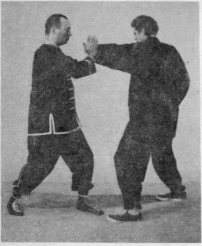

148

147. Right man counters with ram's-head blow.

148. Left man stops intended blow using rock-smash parry.

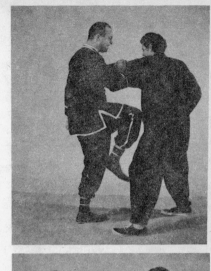

149

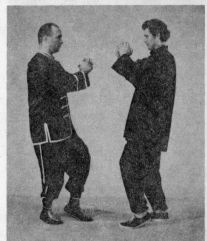

150

149. Left man counters with an elephant kick
(upward with the knee).

150. Both men return to salutation position.

They then return to position of attention.

TIGER FORM

The action in this form is done in a small area.
There is versatility in the hand blows, and movement
toward all the compass points, but relatively little
movement out into the spaces away from the hub of
the action.

151. Assume horse stance.

152. Moving clockwise, step back with your right
foot to face right; deliver rock-smash blow with right
hand.

153. Turning counterclockwise, pivot around to face
left; deliver scorpion blow with right hand.

154. Moving clockwise, step around with left foot
to face front with left foot advanced; deliver tiger-
claw blow with left hand.

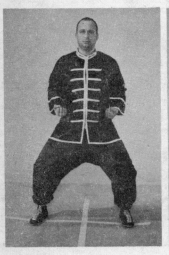 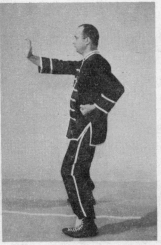

151   152

155. Take short step forward with right foot as you deliver ram's-head blow with right hand.

156. Turning clockwise, step back with your right foot so that you face right; deliver a rock-smash blow with your left hand.

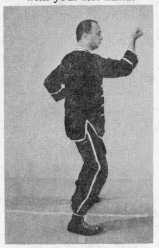

153

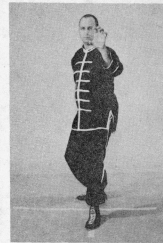

154

155

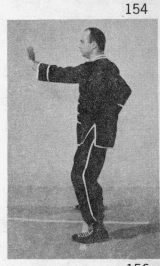

156

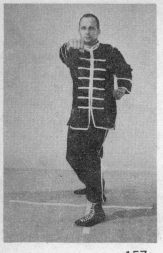 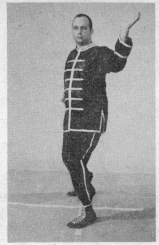

157   158

157. Without moving your feet, turn your body to face front as you deliver ram's-head blow with your right hand.

158. Raise your left hand in knife-slash blow position.

159. Without stepping, pivot on the balls of both feet, turn clockwise to face rear.

160. Without foot movement, deliver knife-slash blow with left hand.

161. Take a step to rear to assume horse stance facing rear; as you step, your left hand simulates grabbing action as your right hand assumes position for delivering rock-smash blow.

162. Deliver rock-smash blow with right hand.

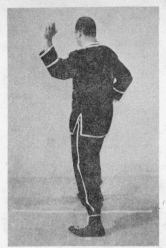

159

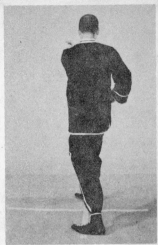

160

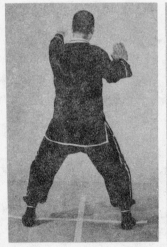

161

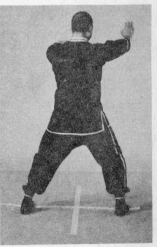

162

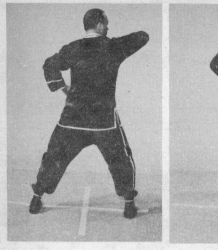 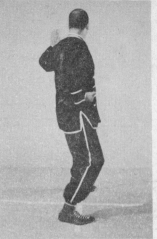

163   164

163. Without foot movement, deliver a monkey blow with right elbow.

164. Take short step to rear with left foot as you deliver rock-smash blow with left hand.

165. Without foot movement, deliver ram's-head punch with right hand.

166. Pivot on right foot, turn clockwise into cat stance facing left with left foot advanced; raise left arm into position for pounding wave blow.

167. Take short step with left foot as you deliver knife-slash blow with left hand.

168. Pivot on left foot, step around counterclockwise with right foot to face rear in horse stance with your fists palm-over-palm at your left hip.

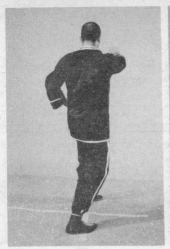
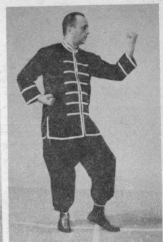

165   166

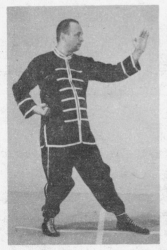

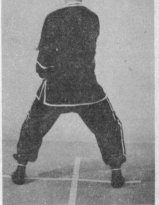

167   168

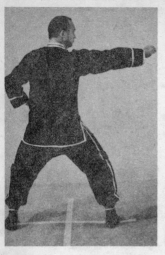 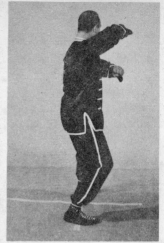

169   170

169. Without foot movement, look left and deliver side hammer blow with your right hand.

170. Pivot on right foot, step to rear with left foot into side horse stance; with both arms in high front guard.

171. Without foot movement, deliver simultaneous blows with both hands; right hand delivers ram's-head blow, left hand delivers side hammer blow.

172. Without foot movement, bring right fist back to hip as left hand delivers rock-smash blow.

173. Turning counterclockwise, take a step back with your left foot to face right in horse stance as you deliver pounding-wave blow with right hand.

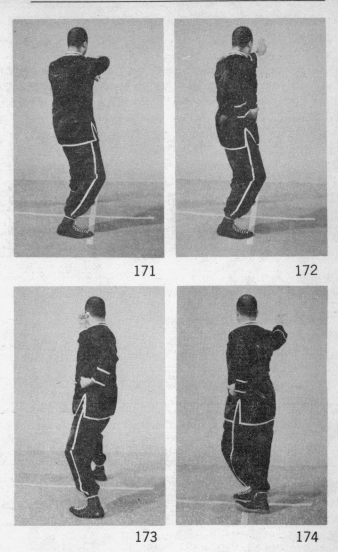

171

172

173

174

174. With your left foot step across your right foot as you deliver whipping-branch block with right hand, palm up.

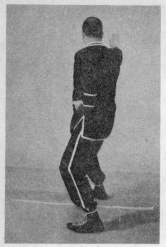 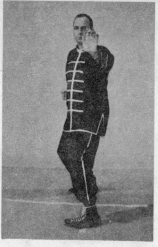

175   176

175. Take a step to rear with right foot to assume horse stance facing right as you deliver rock-smash blow to rear with your right hand.

176. Without foot movement, look front as you deliver rock-smash blow with left hand.

177. With left foot in place, assume cat stance with right foot advanced toward right; right hand is brought to pounding-wave-blow position.

178. Take short step with right foot as you deliver knife-slash blow with left hand.

179. Turning counterclockwise, pivot into horse stance facing front; deliver knife-slash with left hand.

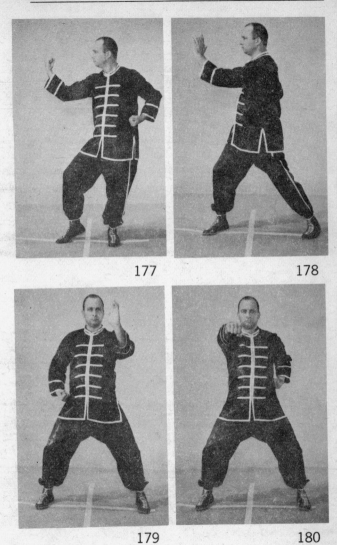

177

178

179

180

180. No foot movement, deliver ram's-head blow with right fist as left fist comes back to hip.

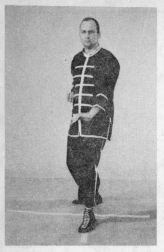
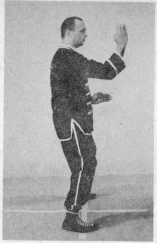

181   182

181. Pivot on right foot, take step to front with left foot as you deliver low knife-slash block with left hand.

182. Moving counterclockwise, pivot on left foot, take a step around with right foot to assume horse stance facing left; raise your right hand in knife-slash blow position.

183. As you whip your right hand back to hip, deliver knife-slash blow with left hand.

184. Without foot movement, turn your body to face front; deliver rock-smash blow with left hand.

185. Without foot movement, draw left hand back and deliver pounding-wave blow with it.

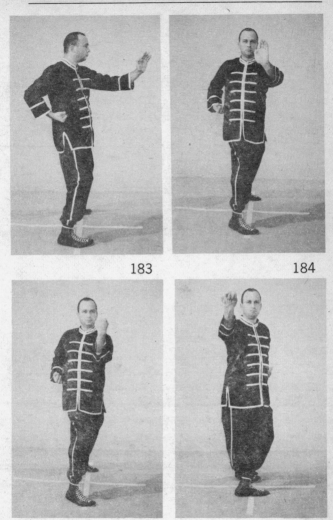

183   184

185   186

186. Step across your right foot with your left foot as you deliver whipping-branch block with right arm, palm up.

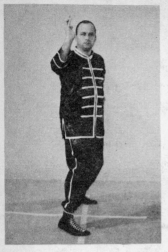 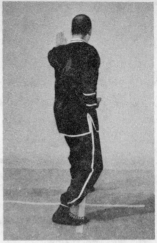

187   188

187. Take step to front with right foot as you deliver knife-slash blow with right hand.

188. Without foot movement, turn your body to face rear as you deliver rock-smash blow with left hand.

189. Moving counterclockwise, step with right foot into horse stance facing rear as you deliver boulder block at head height to left side with your right arm.

190. Without foot movement, twist your body clockwise to left side as you deliver knife-slash with left hand.

191. Moving counterclockwise, step back with left foot into horse stance facing right side; look front as you deliver ram's-head blow to front with right hand.

192. Step with right foot across left foot, fists to hips.

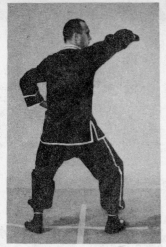

189

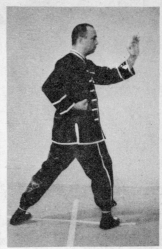

190

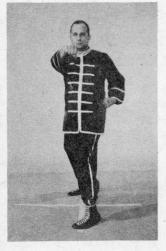

191

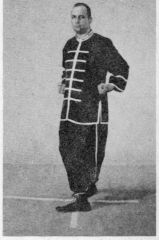

192

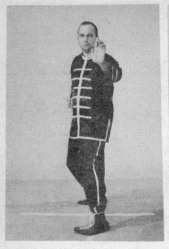 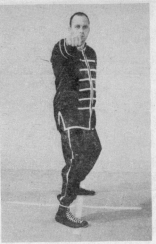

193   194

193. Take step to front with left foot (body faces right side) as you deliver rock-smash blow with left hand.

194. Turning counterclockwise, step around with your right foot into horse stance facing left side; deliver ram's-head blow to front with right hand.

195. Draw right foot back and assume crouching cat stance as your right arm is brought into high guard.

196. Drop into very low crouching cat stance as you deliver pounding-wave blow with right hand.

197. Rise into standing cat stance as you bring your right hand into low guard and your left hand into high guard.

198. Step to front with your left foot.

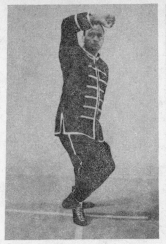

195

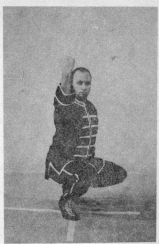

196

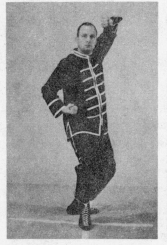

197

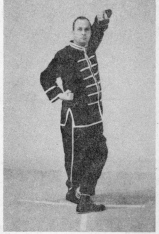

198

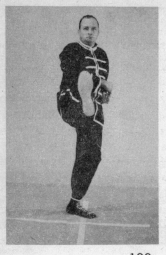 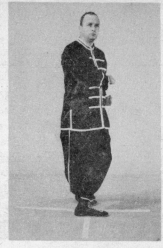

199   200

199. Deliver dragon stamp with your right foot as you bring your fists palm-over-palm at left hip.

200. Your kicking foot is placed down behind your left foot.

201. Pivot on both feet, turning clockwise to assume horse stance facing right side, both hands in high guard.

202. Without foot movement, bring left palm over right fist.

203. No foot movement; in slow motion extend arms fully toward front, in palm-over-fist position.

204. Step back with left foot into position of attention, fists at hips.

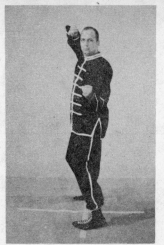

201

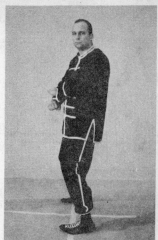

202

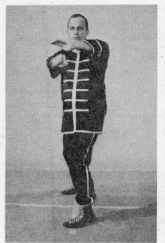

203

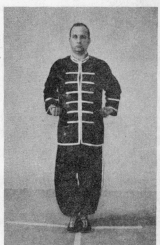

204

EAGLE FORM

The eagle, getting its food, hovers, swoops, dives, grasps and tears. The hand movements, particularly, in this form, imitate gestures which are similar to that of a bird of prey.

Start from the position of attention.

205. Assume a horse stance, facing front.

206-207. Without foot movement, make circular movements with your fists; your left fist moves clockwise, while your right fist moves counterclockwise; make three full revolutions before making the next move.

208. As you step forward with left foot (both feet point right) look front and deliver a rock-smash blow forward with your left hand.

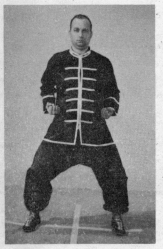
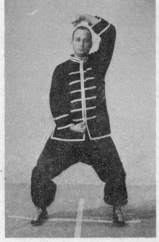

205   206

209. Without drawing your left hand back, move it, fully extended, to right front.

210. Grab and pull with left hand as you deliver scorpion blow with right hand.

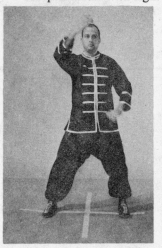

207

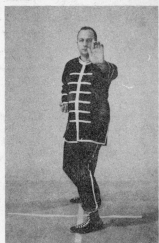

208

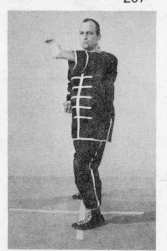

209

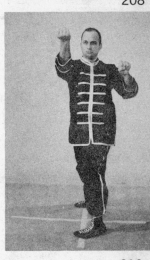

210

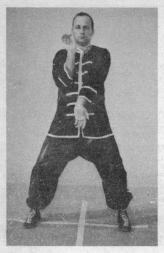 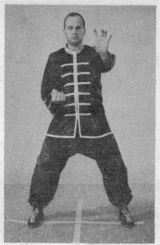

211   212

211. Moving counterclockwise, step around to front with right foot into horse stance and place your hands in open-talon position, elbows in close to your body.

212. As you draw your right fist to hip, your left hand assumes grasping-talon position forward.

213. Bring right fist up toward right shoulder.

214. As your left fist is drawn back to hip, right hand delivers pounding-wave blow forward.

215. Without foot movement, face right as you deliver scorpion blow with right hand toward right side.

216. Moving counterclockwise, step back around with left foot as you raise both arms in high guard.

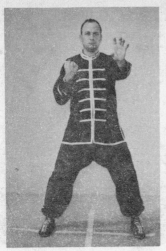

213

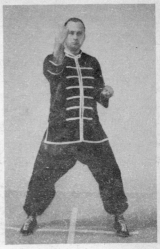

214

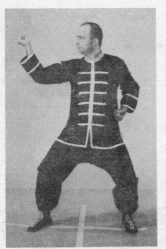

215

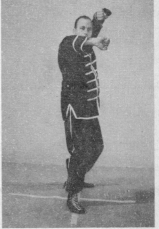

216

217. Moving clockwise, take a step with your left foot into horse stance facing front and make simultaneous hand blows; your left hand delivers tiger-claw blow as your right hand delivers scorpion blow.

218. Without foot movement, twist your body to face left front and deliver knife-slash blow with your right hand.

219. Without foot movement, twist your body to face right front and deliver knife-slash blow with left hand.

220. Without foot movement, face front as your left hand is raised in high guard.

221. As your left fist is brought back to hip, deliver knife-slash forward with right hand.

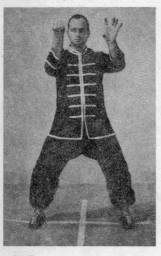
217

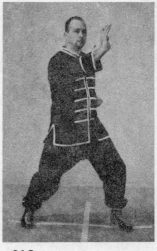
218

222. Moving counterclockwise, step back with left foot to face left as you bring right hand into low knife-slash blow position.

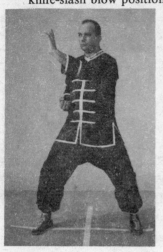
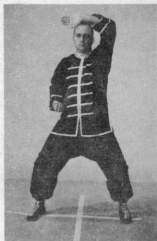

219   220

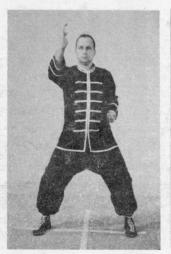
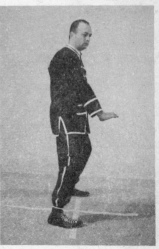

221   222

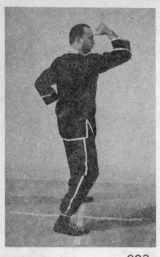 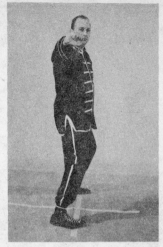

223   224

223. Without foot movement, deliver monkey blow with right elbow.

224. Deliver side hammer blow to front with right hand.

225. Draw right hand inward and then deliver scorpion blow to front.

226. Without foot movement, twist your body toward the front as you deliver rock-smash blow front with your left hand.

227. As you withdraw left hand, deliver pounding-wave blow with right hand.

228. Step with your right foot across left foot toward rear as you deliver scorpion blow rear with your left hand.

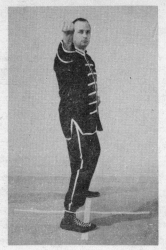

225

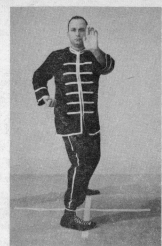

226

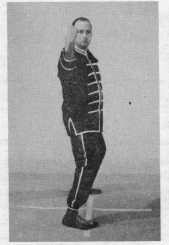

227

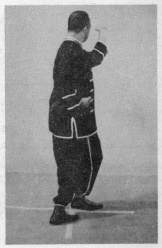

228

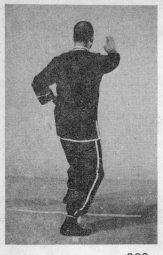 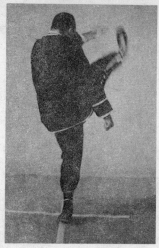

229   230

229. Step to rear with your left foot as you deliver rock-smash blow with right hand.

230. As you deliver dragon stamp to rear with right foot, deliver knife point blow with left hand.

231. As you place your kicking foot down, deliver tiger-claw blow with right hand.

232. Stepping clockwise with your left foot, assume horse stance facing rear.

233. Moving clockwise, step around with your right foot into horse stance facing left side as you deliver boulder block with your right arm.

234. Without foot movement, twist your body to face front and place both hands in open-talon position.

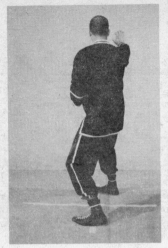

231

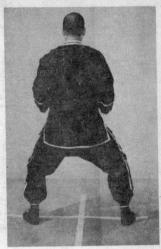

232

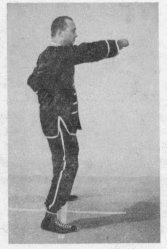

233

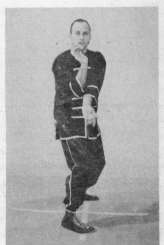

234

235. As you place your fists palm over palm at your left side, deliver dragon stamp to left side with your left foot.

236. Swing your kicking leg around so that you turn counterclockwise to assume horse stance facing rear and deliver pounding-wave blow to left side with your right hand.

237. As you step across your left foot with your right foot, deliver whipping-branch block with your left hand.

238. Take step to right side with your left foot to assume horse stance toward rear; look right and deliver rock-smash blow with right hand.

239. Moving counterclockwise, step around and back with your left foot to assume horse stance facing front; right hand in low guard, left hand in high guard.

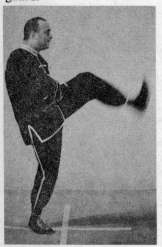
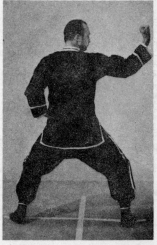

235   236

240. Left foot in place, take short step to right with right foot as you face right and deliver pounding-wave blow with right hand.

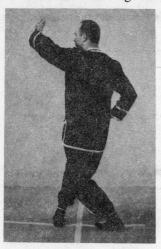
237

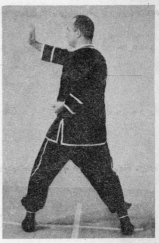
238

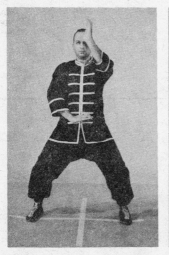
239

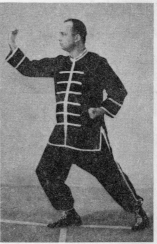
240

241. Moving clockwise pivot on right foot, swing left foot around to face rear; weight is shifted onto your right leg; deliver pounding-wave blow with your left hand.

242. Shift your weight into horse stance as you deliver rock-smash blow with left hand.

243. Moving counterclockwise, pivot on left foot, swing right foot around to assume horse stance facing front; deliver scorpion blow with right hand.

244. No foot movement; look left front as you deliver low knife-slash blow with left hand.

245. No foot movement; look right as you deliver pounding-wave blow with your right hand.

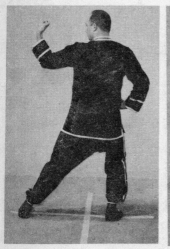
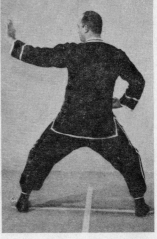

241   242

246. Step to front with your left foot as you place left hand in knife-slash blow position and your right hand makes a tearing-beak action.

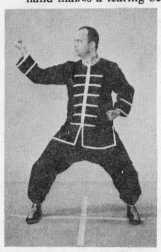

243

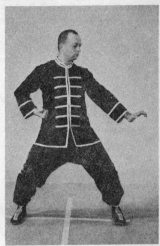

244

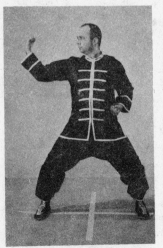

245

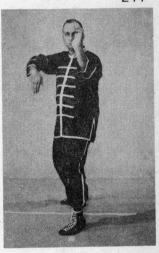

246

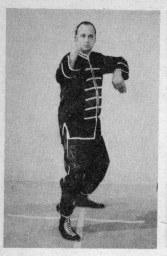
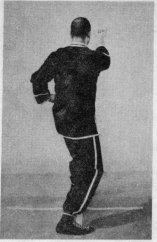

247   248

247. Moving counterclockwise, step to front with right foot as your right hand is placed in knife-slash blow position and your left hand makes a tearing-beak action.

248. Without stepping, pivot to face rear and deliver scorpion blow rear with right hand.

249. Deliver dragon stamp to rear with right foot.

250. As the kicking foot is placed down, make the tearing-beak action with your left hand.

251. Deliver pounding-wave blow to rear with your right hand.

252. Step around clockwise with your left foot into horse stance facing rear.

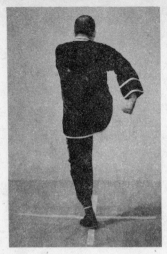

249

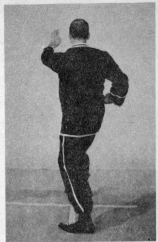

250

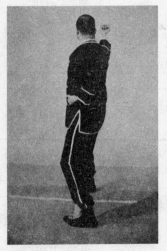

251

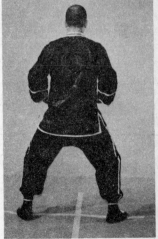

252

253. Deliver knife-slash blow with left hand.

254. Moving clockwise step around and back with your right foot into horse stance facing left side; deliver hammer blow with right hand.

255. Without foot movement, twist your body to face front as you bring both hands into high guard.

256. Place hands in palm over fist position.

257. Extend arms fully toward front.

258. Moving clockwise, step into position of attention with fists at sides.

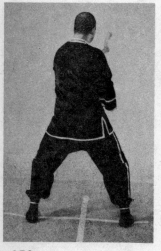

253

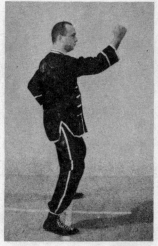

254

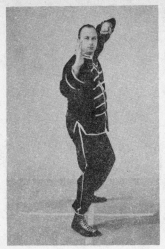

255

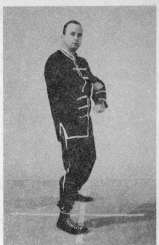

256

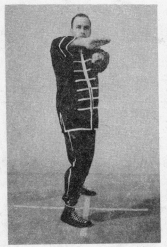

257

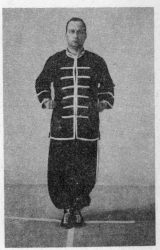

258

TAI CHI

TAI CHI

Tai chi is a splendid exercise. All the movements of
tai chi are natural to the human body and enhance
the normal functions of the human body. Unlike
classical yoga, tai chi does not force the limbs into
grotesque and unnatural postures. In tai chi, all
bending is forward, which is natural for human
anatomy and good for the human spine.

The movements of tai chi involve the whole body,
from head to feet. Coordination is enhanced through
the rhythmic, flowing style of the routine; balance
and body gestures are improved.

Because there is no competition involved, tai chi
promotes a relaxed mental attitude which transfers
to relax the body. No special apparatus is needed
and it is a solo routine, which can be done almost
anywhere at the time of day convenient and pleasant
for the person doing it.

Coordination of eye-limb activity involves a degree
of mental concentration which is stimulating and
relaxing. Flexibility, grace and lightness of movement, and emotional refreshment can result from
earnest and diligent practice of tai chi.

Although there are no reliable written records of the
history of tai chi, there are enough fragments of
evidence to indicate that it originated as an exercise to maintain agility and perfect the gestures of
kung fu karate. It was practiced by Chinese kung fu
fighters in the feudal period and was the equivalent
of shadow-boxing.

From its original form, which had only the purpose of training fighters, tai chi developed two distinct styles, with many substyles arising from them. The two principal styles were hard-style and soft-style tai chi. Hard-style tai chi is vigorous and imitates the fighting gestures of kung fu hand and foot blows; the soft style has evolved into an exercise in which the hand and foot movements hardly resemble the original hitting and kicking actions.

Tai chi is a valuable exercise with many legitimate benefits. But tai chi has been extravagantly praised as the "ultimate," the "divine," the "supreme" exercise and claims have been made for the therapeutic value of tai chi. For this reason, we ought to examine tai chi in terms of modern physiological knowledge and in terms of modern developments in physical education.

Perhaps in the time when tai chi was developed, for a class of people who did absolutely no exercise at all, nor any physical labor, tai chi was indeed the ultimate in physical exercise.

For their time, the ancient Chinese were very advanced in knowledge; compared with what we know today about anatomy and body function, they knew very little.

Their evaluation of tai chi, while valid for their time, their culture and their needs is not valid for our time and culture. A new evaluation which assigns tai chi its proper place is necessary. Tai chi, while promoting the important elements of flexibility, coordination, poise and balance, lacks an essential which might qualify it as the "only" exercise; in tai chi there is no vigor, not enough heart-lung stimulation now known to be essential in maintaining good body function. If you are aged or infirm, or convalescent, then tai chi might be the only effective exercise you can do and tai chi could confer on you all the benefits of exercise which you are capable of doing. Unless you are aged or infirm, you should include in your program energetic exercise to round out and complete the benefits which you derive from tai chi. Walking-jogging, swimming, handball, tennis — anything which promotes cardio-vascular stimulation will do. The kung fu form, if done with maximum vigor, could be the complementary activity to give you a complete exercise program.

In China today, tai chi is widely practiced, but it is not the only exercise they do. The Chinese people engage in many vigorous exercises.

As for the therapeutic claims made for tai chi — they are misleading. Tai chi promoters claim that tai chi exercise will cure as many diseases and restore as many non-functioning organs as the old snake-oil remedies. While it is true that practice of the routine will promote general health and you will feel better if you do tai chi, there is absolutely no acceptable evidence that tai chi is a substitute for medical care. A tai chi teacher is without any preparation for diagnosing disease, or for prescribing for cure or care. If you are ill, see a doctor. If your ailment could be "cured" by doing tai chi, it could be "cured" by any routine of exercise. It is a cruel deception to make promises of "cure"; rather than enhancing the reputation of tai chi, it lowers it to the rank of a quack or crank activity. Tai chi is a good exercise and it deserves to be rescued from the bad reputation of cure-all quackery.

AWARENESS AND MOVEMENT

It is possible to memorize a series of physical actions
and then do them in an absent-minded fashion; we
do routine physical things absent-mindedly all the
time. The purpose of tai chi is to make certain that
the mind is present, not absent, during the performance of the movements.

Awareness and concentration are not mysterious
functions; they are functions which you control. As
you make each move, think about it; let your mind
dwell on the form, the shape, the body posture.
Awareness is involvement of the conscious senses
and being aware of what you are doing, whether it is
tai chi, brushing your teeth or running along the
beach, makes you feel more alive than doing things
mechanically. So, you begin the tai chi exercises by
being aware of yourself doing tai chi. As you progress,
you can develop more and more awareness, which
will give you increasing vitality and satisfaction.

The practice of tai chi should be undertaken as an
enjoyable activity. There cannot be strain or forcing,
either in the physical actions or in your mental
approach to learning and practicing tai chi. As the
movements are gentle, flowing, rounded and smooth,
so must your mind accept the activity of tai chi in a
gentle, non-resisting manner. Do not practice tai
chi as a duty; practice tai chi as a creative experience
of mind and body.

Because none of the tai chi movements themselves
are difficult to perform, the routine lends itself to
this gentle approach. This is not to say that learning
and doing tai chi is without difficulty; it requires

attention and involvement to memorize the routine, but it does not require struggle. If you find yourself struggling to learn the movements and fighting with yourself to do them, you should retreat and start again.

STYLE OF MOVEMENT IN TAI CHI

Tai chi movements are slow, smooth, rounded, flowing, gentle. There is no perceptible hesitation between the postures after they have been learned.

Rounded, curling gestures prevail in tai chi. Even when the final gesture is straight forward, it is usually preceded by a rounded movement, or a sweeping, curling of the hands or arms.

Steps are taken very lightly and softly. Feel yourself "floating" through the actions as though you were floating in air or making the gestures in water. Think through the idea of moving in water and you will get a very good mental image of a good style of practicing tai chi. When you move in water, if you move very slowly and do not fight the water, your movements are slow, langorous, easy; if you push and fight the water, your movements will be floundering, clumsy, difficult. Keep the image of slow gentle movements, smooth as a bird in the air, smooth as sea grass in water.

Do not worry too much about little variations of posture; the main thing is to capture the attitude and essence of the movements. If you do that, you get the benefits of the exercise.

GREAT CIRCLE

259. Standing repose, face the east.

260. The breath comes in as arms rise . . .

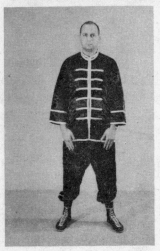

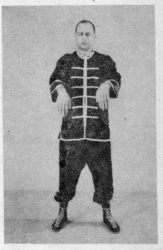

259   260

261. . . . to reach the chest height as full breath is taken in the body . . .

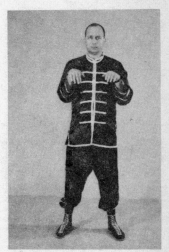

261

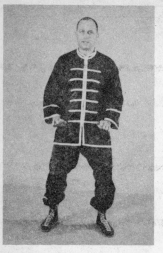 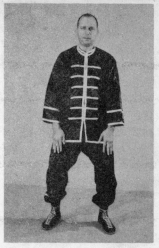

262   263

262. . . . and the breath begins to leave as the arms continue the flowing motion downward . . .

263. . . . to reach the thighs as the knees are bent slightly to assume quarter-squat position with a straight back.

264. TOUCH THE SOUTH WIND. As the body turns to the south with weight lightly placed on right foot (left foot remains in place), the hands move as though around the rim of a large circle with the left hand at the top of the rim.

265. The hands continue to move around the rim of the circle until the left hand falls off the rim, palm back, and the right hand, reaching the top of the rim pushes gently forward into the wind, palm toward face. As the right hand rises, so does the right foot . . .

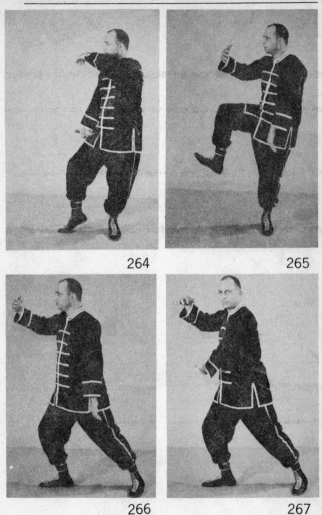

264

265

266

267

266. . . . and the motion continues as the right foot is placed down and body weight is shifted forward.

267. TOUCH THE EAST WIND. As the hands come back to the rim of the wheel (right hand high) the head turns to look at the east . . .

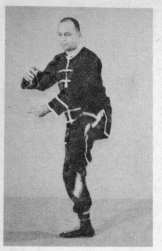 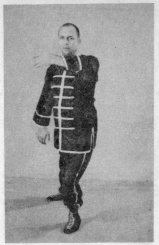

268   269

268. . . . and the left leg is raised as the hands move around the rim . . .

269. . . . and left foot is placed down, bearing weight, with the right hand falling off the rim at the low point (palm back), as the left hand pushes gently forward against the wind, palm toward face.

270. THE TIDE COMES IN AND OUT. As the hands come back to touch the rim of the circle (left hand high), the left foot pivots in place and the body is facing south.

271. Now rim of the wheel is imagined to become very small to bring the hands together high, as the right foot is placed forward, bearing weight.

272. The hands are moved around the rim of the small circle so that the left hand is palm up, as weight leaves the right foot and is shifted back onto the left foot . . .

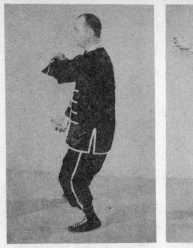
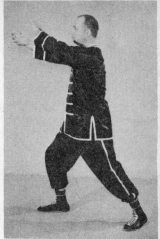

270

271

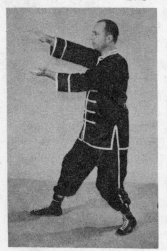
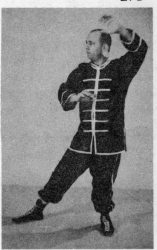

272

273

273. . . . continuing until the weight is fully onto
the left foot and left leg is bent; the hands leave the
circle rim, left hand placed high, palm out and right
hand at chest, palm down.

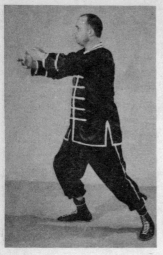 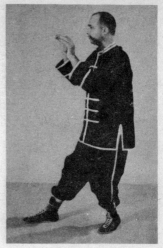

274   275

274. Both hands flow forward, palms together; weight is shifted forward onto right foot.

275. Arms flow back, palms out, as weight is shifted back onto left foot.

276. Arms flow forward, palm out, as weight shifts forward onto right foot.

277. THE CRANE. As the upper body turns to the north, the arms flow around, palms down, feet pivot in place, beginning a counterclockwise turn.

278. As the turn is completed and body faces north, the left leg is raised with heel at knee; arms flow up with right hand drooped, shoulder height, left hand pushes gently forward, palm away from face, 279.

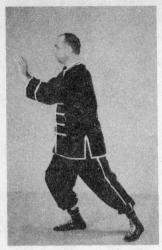

276

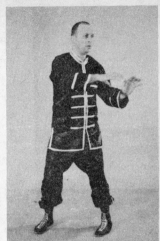

277

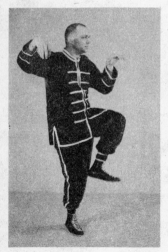

278

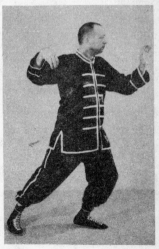

279

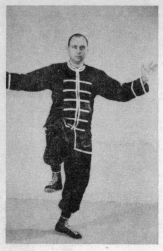 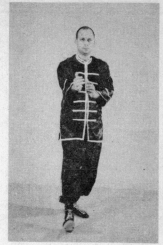

280   281

280. BIRD PERCHING. Body is turned to face east, as both arms make wide, flowing circle and right knee is raised.

281. Raised foot is placed forward upon the heel as both hands come close together.

282. Weight of the body shifts forward as right foot rocks from heel to toe; both arms flow toward northwest.

283. Right foot makes slight step forward and body weight shifts to follow it; left hand clasps right wrist and both arms sway slightly forward.

284. VIEW TO THE NORTH. As the body is turned to face north, left foot is placed forward lightly; left arm hangs loosely at the side, right hand moves up to head height and is held palm down.

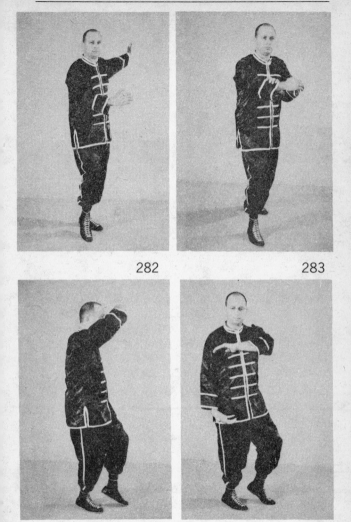

282

283

284

285

285. TAKE PATH TO LEFT. As the body is turned
to the east, both arms flow around and hands are
placed as though on the rim of the large circle, right
hand at the bottom of the rim.

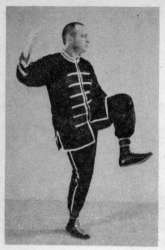 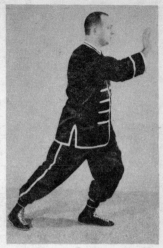

286   287

286. As the hands move around the rim of the circle to bring the right hand to the top of the rim, the left foot takes a high step; as the left hand reaches the bottom of the rim of the circle, it drops away to the side; body is twisted to face north.

287. The stepping foot is placed down and the body weight shifts toward it as the right hand presses gently forward, palm away from face.

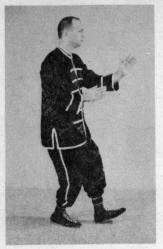 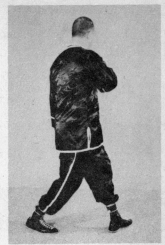

288   289

288. READY WITH STAFF. As the body weight flows back onto the right foot and left heel, the right hand flows down and back and around the rim of a small circle as the left hand flows up and around the rim until both hands are in the staff-holding pose.

Repeat the movements of TAKE PATH TO LEFT, photos 285-287.

289. TAKE PATH TO RIGHT. As body is moved to face west, hands are placed on the rim of the circle, right hand at the top.

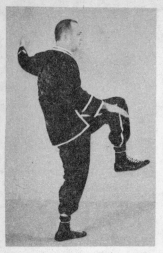
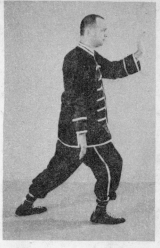

290   291

290. As body turns back to face north, the hands are moved around the rim to place the left hand high; the right foot takes a high step as the right hand drops off the bottom of the rim.

291. The stepping foot is placed down and the body weight shifts toward it, as the left hand presses gently forward, palm away from face.

Repeat TAKE PATH TO LEFT, photos 285-287.

Repeat READY WITH STAFF, photo 288.

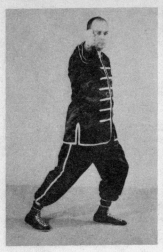
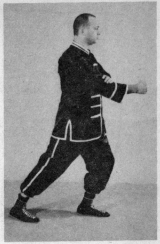

292   293

Repeat TAKE PATH TO LEFT, photos 285-287.

292. STRONG RIGHT FIST. As the right hand is pulled back and under the rim of a circle it forms a fist and then moves over the top of the rim of a circle toward the east.

293. FACE THE WIND. The right fist is drawn back and close to the right side as the right foot takes a step to the north; the right fist moves along a straight line directly forward as the left hand clasps the right upper arm and the left foot takes a step with the body weight flowing forward.

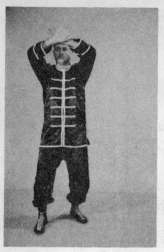 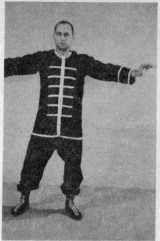

294   295

294. THE SUN WHEEL. Body is turned to face east as the hands describe outward circles bringing them up to the head, palms away from face.

295. Flowing hands move outward, palms down . . .

296. . . . and continue sweeping movement to crossed position at chest, palms in . . .

297. . . . and drop gently at thighs, palms in.

298. PART THE SOUTH WIND. Right foot glides to south as body weight shifts onto left foot.

299. Right foot steps high as left hand sweeps up to shoulder height.

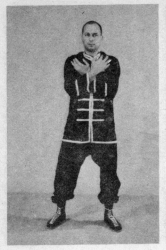

296

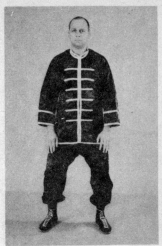

297

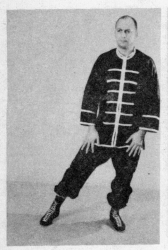

298

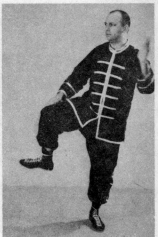

299

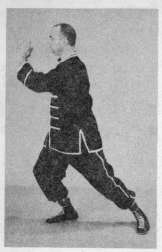
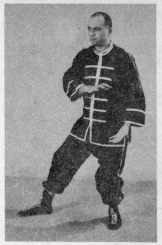

300   301

300. As stepping foot is placed down and body weight shifts onto it, left hand moves gently toward the south, edge of hand forward.

301. GRASP THE WHEEL. As body weight shifts back onto left foot, the hands flow around in position to hold the rim of a circle, right hand at chest height, left hand low.

Repeat THE TIDE COMES IN AND OUT, photos 270-276.

Repeat THE CRANE, photos 277, 278.

302. BIRD WITH FOLDED WING. As the right foot steps forward and the body weight flows with it, left arm flows back and is placed at spine, as right arm curves forward and is placed at chest height, hands loose.

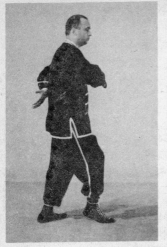

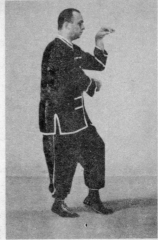

302   303

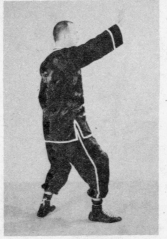

304

303. As left foot is moved forward, bearing light weight, left arm circles around into bird beak; right hand becomes loose fist.

304. RECEDING WAVES. Step back with left foot as right arm rises gently and left arm drops down to the side, palm forward.

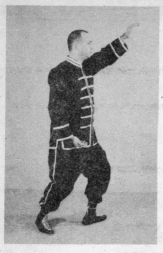 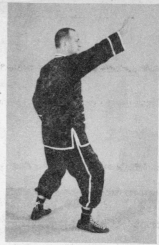

305   306

305. Step back with the right foot as left arm rises gently and right arm falls down to the side, palm forward.

306. Repeat the movement of photo 304.

307. TURNING THE WHEEL. Without foot movement, both hands grasp lightly, as though holding the rim of a large wheel, left hand at the top of the rim.

308. As the hands turn the wheel so that the right hand holds it gently out and forward, the body is turned toward the east, right foot forward.

Repeat BIRD PERCHING, photos 280-283.

Repeat VIEW TO THE NORTH, photo 284.

Repeat TAKE PATH TO LEFT, photos 285-287.

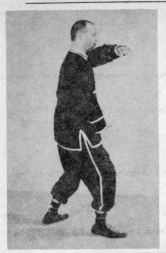
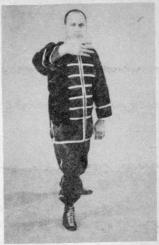

307   308

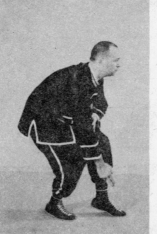

309

309. TAKE THE BLOSSOM. As the right foot takes
one short step forward followed by a short step forward with the left foot, the body gently lowers with
a curling of the back and bending of the knees; right
hand is drawn back then placed near the left foot,
left hand sweeps across and the fingers lightly touch
at right elbow.

310. PRAISE THE NORTH. As the body rises slowly to standing, weight mainly on right foot, both arms fold toward the chest, hands held palm out.

311. As left foot steps forward and body weight is shifted onto it, both hands are extended forward, palms out.

312. REAPING WIND. As the body turns to face south, weight kept on left foot, right arm folds into chest, then makes loose fist, extends and wheels out as left hand drops to side.

313. FACE THE WIND, SOUTH. Step around with left foot to face south with left foot forward, repeat arm movement of FACE THE WIND, photo 293.

Repeat GRASP THE WHEEL, photo 301.

Repeat THE TIDE COMES IN AND OUT, photos 270-276.

Repeat THE CRANE, photos 277-278.

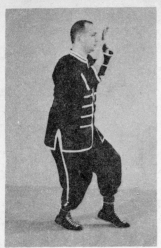

310

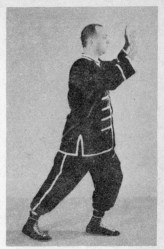

311

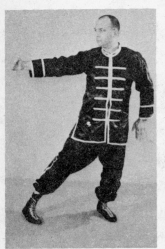

312

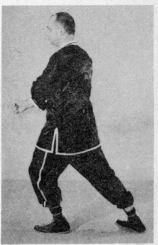

313

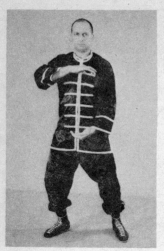
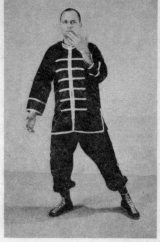

314   315

314. WINGS OPEN AND CLOSE. Turn on the balls of both feet to face east as the hands assume position of lightly grasping the large wheel, right hand on top of the rim.

315. A short step forward is taken with the left foot, the left hand flows upward with palm toward face, as right hand flows downward.

316. As short step is taken with right foot, right hand flows up and left hand flows down.

Repeat THE CRANE, photos 277, 278.

317. PART THE NORTH WIND. Both hands fold into chest and then press gently forward, palms out.

318. As the body weight is shifted back on the right foot, right hand drops gently down to side, palm up.

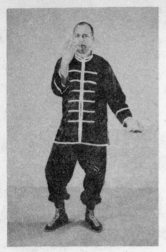

316

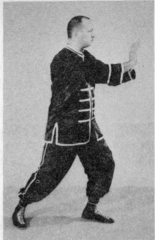

317

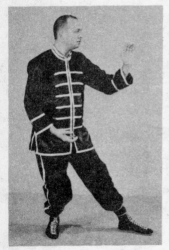

318

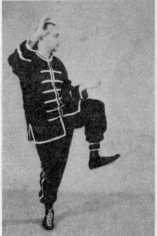

319

319. As both hands move around the rim of a wheel to bring right hand high, left foot is raised.

320. As the left foot is placed down and body weight shifts onto it, both hands push gently forward, palms out.

321. DANCING BEAR. As the arms flow outward extended to sides, right leg is raised and then extended.

322. As the right foot is placed down and body weight shifts onto it, both arms wave inward and then outward as left leg is raised and then extended.

Turn to face south and repeat 322.

Repeat TAKE PATH TO LEFT, photos 285-287.

Repeat TAKE PATH TO RIGHT, photos 289-291.

Pivot to face south.

323. DEFY THE DRAGON. As a step is taken forward with the left foot, right hand assumes loose fist position, circles at the side and then extends forward with elbow bent; left hand swoops over to touch lightly at right elbow.

Step around with left foot to face north

Repeat DEFY THE DRAGON, photo 323.

Repeat REAPING WIND, photo 312.

Repeat FACE THE WIND, photo 313.

Repeat DANCING BEAR, photos 321, 322.

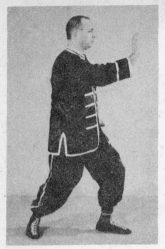

320

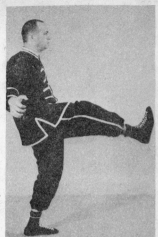

321

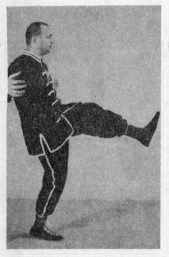

322

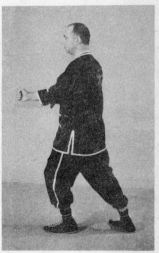

323

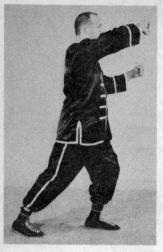
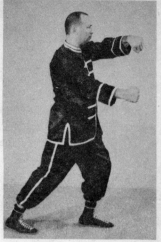

324   325

324. **DEFY THE LEOPARD.** As the kicking foot is placed down in back of left foot, body weight shifts onto the left foot; both hands grasp as though holding a thick staff lightly at the left side of the body.

325. The staff is moved from the left to the right side of the body.

326. The staff is pressed forward and upward.

327. **DEFY THE PANTHER.** As a step is taken forward with the right foot and body weight shifted onto it, the staff is placed at chest height.

328. The staff is turned toward the left side of the body.

329. The staff is pushed forward and upward.

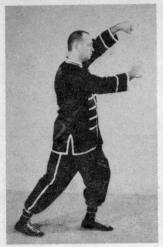
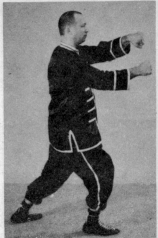

326   327

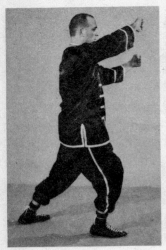
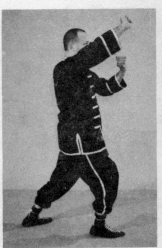

328   329

Repeat DANCING BEAR, photos 321, 322.

330. GRASP THE OARS. As the kicking foot is lowered, the arms swoop inward . . .

331. . . . and as the kicking foot is placed forward and body weight shifted onto it, the hands grasp as though holding oars.

Repeat DANCING BEAR using left foot, as in photo 322.

Repeat GRASP THE OARS, photos 330, 331.

Repeat DANCING BEAR using left foot, photos 321, 322.

Repeat TAKE PATH TO LEFT, photos 285, 287.

Repeat STRONG RIGHT FIST, photo 292.

Repeat FACE THE WIND, photo 313.

Repeat THE SUN WHEEL, photos 294-297.

Repeat PART THE SOUTH WIND, photos 298-300.

Repeat GRASP THE WHEEL, photo 301.

Repeat THE TIDE COMES IN AND OUT, photos 270-276.

Repeat THE CRANE, photos 277, 278.

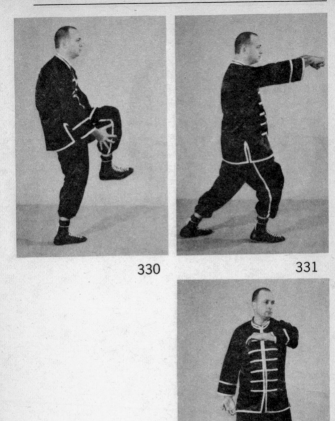

330

331

332

332. PLACING THE SHIELD RIGHT. Shifting to face northeast, place hands lightly as though holding a curved shield; place left arm into the shield at chest height.

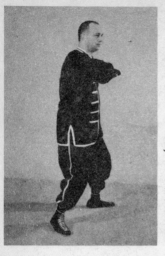 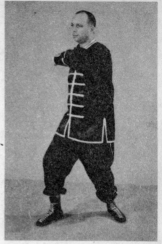

333   334

333. As left arm flows down to the side, right arm is placed into the shield at chest height, as body shifts to face north.

334. Without stepping, pivot and turn body to face southeast as right hand drops to side and left arm is placed in shield.

335. Without stepping, body weight flows back to shift onto left foot as both hands grasp small sphere, right hand on top.

336. Turn the sphere so that left hand is at the top.

337. As right foot takes step forward, left hand drops to side and right hand is held shoulder height, palm toward face.

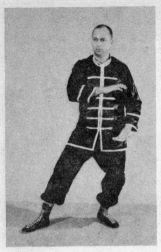

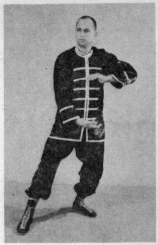

335 336

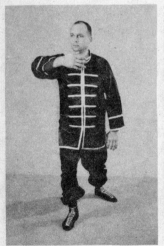

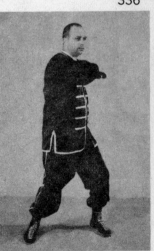

337 338

338. PLACING THE SHIELD LEFT. Without stepping, twist the body to face northeast as right arm is placed in shield at chest height and left hand drops to side.

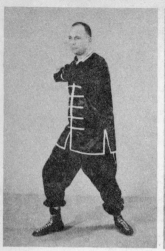
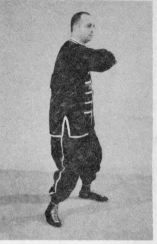

339   340

339. Without stepping, pivot and turn body toward southeast as right hand drops to side and left arm is placed in shield.

340. Without stepping, body twists to face northeast as left hand drops to side and right arm is placed in shield.

341. As step is taken back with right foot, both hands grasp sphere lightly, left hand at the top.

342. Without foot movement, sphere is rotated so the right hand is at the top.

343. As left foot takes step to northeast, right hand drops to side and left arm is placed shoulder height, palm toward face.

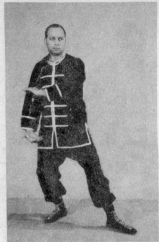

341

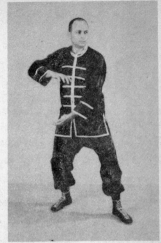

342

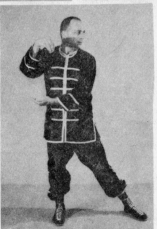

343

Repeat PLACING THE SHIELD RIGHT, photos 332-337.

Repeat TOUCH THE SOUTH WIND, photos 264-266.

Repeat THE TIDE COMES IN AND OUT, photos 270-276.

Repeat THE CRANE, photos 277, 278.

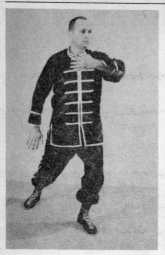 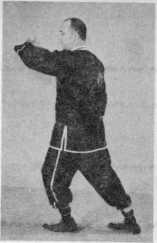

344   345

344. **DARK LADY SPINS FLAX.** Body weight is shifted onto right leg; left leg is extended and bears little weight; left hand is placed at right side, palm up.

345. Step around with left foot to face south as right hand drops to right side and left hand comes up to head height, palm toward face.

346. Right foot steps behind left foot, weight placed lightly on tip of right foot as right palm touches left forearm.

347. Weight flows back onto right foot as right hand drops to waist height, palm up.

348. Right foot makes step toward north to place body facing west, as left hand drops to side and right hand is placed at chest height with palm toward face; right hand presses gently toward north.

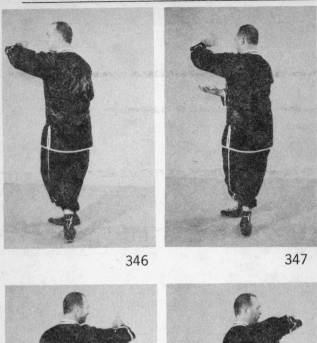

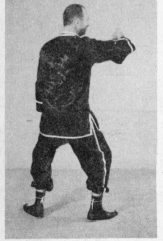

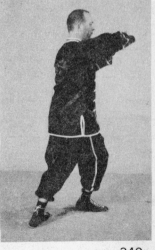

349. Left foot steps behind right foot as left palm is placed at right forearm.

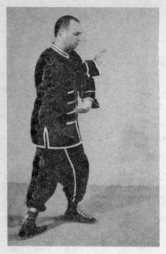
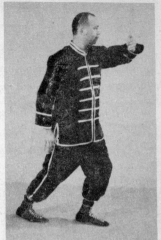

350   351

350. Weight is shifted onto left foot as left hand is placed at waist height, palm down.

351. Step around with left foot to face north as left hand comes up to face height, palm in; right hand drops to right side.

352. Right foot steps behind left foot as right palm is placed at left forearm.

353. Right hand drops to waist height, palm up.

354. Right foot steps to south as right hand is placed head high, palm toward face; left hand drops to side.

355. Left foot steps behind right foot as left palm is placed at right forearm.

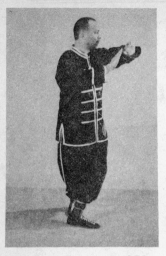

352

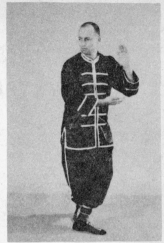

353

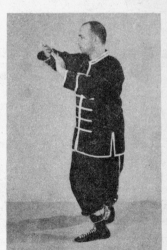

354 355

Left foot takes step back; repeat TOUCH THE EAST WIND, photos 267-269.

Repeat THE TIDE COMES IN AND OUT, photos 270-276.

Repeat THE CRANE, photos 277, 278.

Repeat WINGS OPEN AND CLOSE, photos 314-316.

Repeat THE CRANE, photos 277, 278.

356. SERPENT DESCENDS. Weight shifts back onto bent right leg and then body curls forward as left hand slides down the left leg.

357. THE STORK. As you rise, lift the right leg, knee bent, as the right hand is raised to face height, fingers spread, and left hand drops to side.

358. Right foot is placed down behind left foot and left leg is raised, knee bent, as right hand drops to side and left hand is raised, fingers spread.

Step back with left foot, then repeat RECEDING WAVES, photos 304-306.

Repeat TURNING THE WHEEL, photos 307, 308.

Repeat BIRD PERCHING, photos 280-283.

Repeat VIEW TO THE NORTH, photo 284.

Repeat TAKE PATH TO LEFT, photos 285-287.

Repeat TAKE THE BLOSSOM, photo 309.

Repeat PRAISE THE NORTH, photos 310, 311.

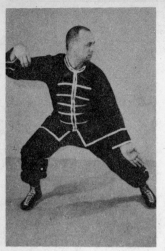

356

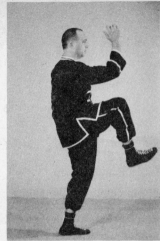

357

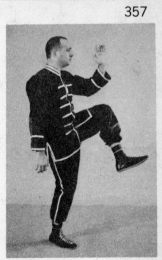

358

Repeat PLACING THE SHIELD RIGHT, photos 332-337.

Repeat TOUCH THE SOUTH WIND, photos 264-266.

359. DRAGON FLAME. Wrists are crossed.

360. Pivot to face south, weight on left leg, as hands flow into sphere-holding position at waist and chest height, left hand at top.

361. As step is taken with right foot, and body weight shifts onto it, arms extend and the sphere becomes smaller.

Take step with left foot and repeat FACE THE WIND, photo 313.

Repeat GRASP THE WHEEL, photo 301.

Repeat THE TIDE COMES IN AND OUT, photos 270-276.

Repeat THE CRANE, photos 277, 278.

Repeat WINGS OPEN AND CLOSE, photos 314-316.

Repeat THE CRANE, photos 277, 278.

Repeat PART THE NORTH WIND, photos 317-320.

362. SUPPLICATION. Weight flows back onto right leg which is bent, as hands flow back to hold small sphere at waist and chest height, left hand at the top.

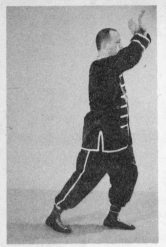

359

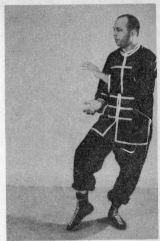

360

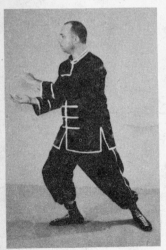

361

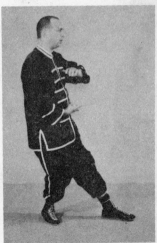

362

363. As weight flows forward onto left bent leg, hands reach forward.

364. Weight shifts back onto right foot as left foot draws toward right foot; tip of left shoe barely touches floor; wrists are crossed at chest, palms toward chest.

Repeat DANCING BEAR using left foot, photos 321, 322.

Repeat TAKE PATH TO LEFT, photos 285-287.

Repeat TAKE PATH TO RIGHT, photos 289-291.

Repeat DEFY THE DRAGON, photo 323.

Repeat GRASP THE WHEEL, photo 301.

Repeat THE TIDE COMES IN AND OUT, photos 270-276.

Repeat THE CRANE, photos 277, 278.

Repeat SERPENT DESCENDS, photo 356.

365. CROSSED BRANCHES. As body rises, weight is shifted to left foot; take step with right foot and cross wrists out in front of your chest, hands are loosely fisted.

Repeat DANCING BEAR using right foot, photos 321, 322.

Repeat VIEW TO THE NORTH, photo 284.

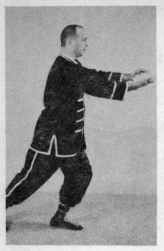

363

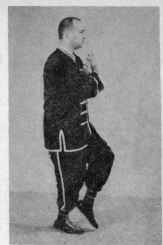

364

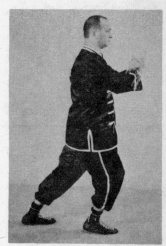

365

Repeat DANCING BEAR using left foot, photos
321, 322.

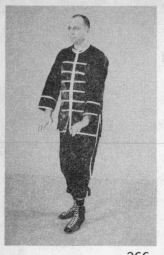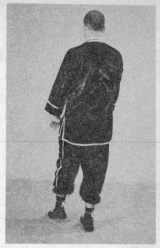

366   367

366. REACHING FOR LIMB. As the left foot is placed down, the arms wave inward.

367. Keeping the right foot in place, pivot on it and turn to face east, then south, then west, then north; you have made a full circle.

368. Shift weight to left leg; extend and raise the right leg and reach toward the right foot with both hands.

Place right foot down forward, shift weight onto it and repeat DEFY THE PANTHER, photos 327-329.

Repeat STRONG RIGHT FIST, photo 292.

Repeat FACE THE WIND, photo 313.

Repeat THE SUN WHEEL, photos 294-297.

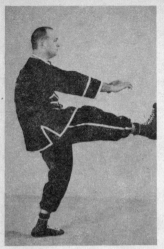

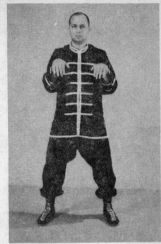

368

369

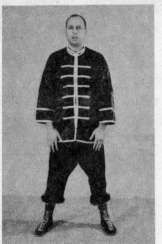

370

369. CONCLUSION. Raise the hands to chest height, wrists limp.

370. Lower hands to hang loosely at thighs.

INDEX

TAI CHI INDEX

Wheel, 156

View to the north, 150

Wings open and close, 164

Strong right fist, 155
Supplication, 182

Take the blossom, 161